**ENT Practice
for the
GP's Surgery**

ENT Practice
for the
GP's Surgery

Andrew N. Coley MB ChB
General Practitioner and Clinical Assistant in Otolaryngology
The Chestnuts Surgery, Poynton, Cheshire, UK

Nicholas J. Kay FRCSEng
Consultant Otolaryngologist,
Stockport Infirmary, Cheshire, UK

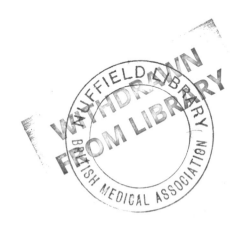

CHURCHILL LIVINGSTONE
EDINBURGH LONDON MADRID MELBOURNE NEW YORK AND TOKYO 1992

CHURCHILL LIVINGSTONE
Medical Division of Longman Group UK Limited

Distributed in the United States of America by
Churchill Livingstone Inc., 650 Avenue of the Americas, New York,
NY 10011, and by associated companies, branches and
representatives throughout the world.

First Published 1992

ISBN 0-443-04813-4

British Library Cataloguing in Publication Data
A catalogue record for this book is available from the British Library

Library of Congress Cataloging in Publication Data available

The
publisher's
policy is to use
paper manufactured
from sustainable forests

Printed in Hong Kong
LYP/01

Preface

ENT problems, especially those in childhood, represent a high percentage of a GP's work load. Unfortunately, there is often little teaching in this subject; as a medical student, this amounts to one or two weeks during five years. Many doctors enter their trainee year with a large void in their knowledge of ENT problems.

Scanty teaching in otolaryngology has resulted in many general practitioners referring patients to hospital out-patient departments far sooner than they would prefer. A wider understanding of the history, examination and management of ENT problems may well result in GPs treating more of their patients within the surgery.

We have strenuously avoided the temptation of producing another comprehensive ENT textbook which, in general practice, would not really be useful. The topics cover the commonly presenting problems and their management in general practice and the text is, therefore, not a comprehensive account of specialist otolaryngology. Examination skills are only those used already and the equipment is no more than can be found in an average GP's surgery.

We feel that this book will be a useful addition to an individual practitioner's reference book collection. The format has been arranged to produce a 'user-friendly' guide, hopefully well-illustrated, to reduce the presence of text which takes time to read. It aims to offer a combination of easy reference and light reading when considering the common presenting ENT symptoms encountered in general practice. The chapters are arranged in such a way as to highlight areas quickly where:

- referral should be automatic
- management within the practice is appropriate and cost-effective
- useful management plans can be made for the middle ground between treatment and referral.

We hope this book will also become an asset in the general practice trainee year, encouraging useful discussion between trainer and trainee. For well-informed trainees to become competent and experienced principals, management of ENT problems will follow a sensible and well-thought out pattern.

This information may also encourage discussion between general practice principals and their local ENT consultants. This can only be beneficial and should improve patient care.

Stockport   A.N.C.
1992   N.J.K.

Acknowledgements

We are indebted to Carolyn Saunders for invaluable skills and willingness in preparing the manuscript.

Our thanks are due to Dr John Sandars for his early encouragement and advice. Our thanks are due also to Abacus Studios (Stockport) for their photographic support. Janssen Pharmaceutical also provided support in the early stages; we are grateful.

Stockport

1992

A.N.C

N.J.K

Illustration acknowledgements

Figures: 2.4, 3.1A (5.3B), 3.1B (5.3E), 3.1C (5.3C), 3.1D (5.1), 3.2A, 3.2B, 3.3, 3.4, 3.6, 3.8, 4.1, 4.2, 4.4A (10.1B), 4.4B (10.1A), 4.5A, 4.5B, 5.3F. Hawke M et al 1990 Clinical Otoscopy: an introduction to ear diseases (2nd end). Churchill Livingstone, Edinburgh. Reproduced with permission of the authors and publishers.

Figures: 3.5 (4.3), 3.7, 10.2, 13.1, 13.4B, 14.1, 16.1, 20.1. Stafford ND and Youngs R 1988 Colour aids: ENT. Churchill Livingstone, Edinburgh. Reproduced with permission of the authors and publishers.

Figures: 12.1, 16.2, 13.3 by courtesy of Mr N Stafford, London.

To our wives, Barbara and Ingrid.

Contents

1. Equipment: basic requirements

The following equipment is recommended, most of which can be found in the GP's bag; the extras should not strain the practice budget.

EARS

- *Otoscope*: it is most useful to have an otoscope with a swinging or sliding lens.

- *Tuning fork*: a 512 Hz fork (Fig. 1.1) with a sounding plate is the most desirable of the range; lower frequencies will be confused by the patient because of vibro-tactile sensation; a higher frequency will decay too quickly to enable a Rinné's test to be effective.

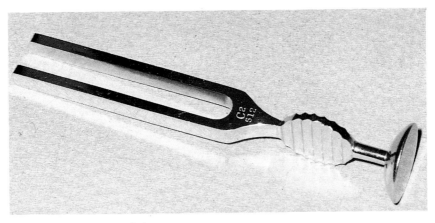

Fig. 1.1   A 512 Hz tuning fork.

- *Ear syringe*: the classical metal design is adequate (Fig. 1.2), but automatically pressured pumps (Fig. 1.3) are also relatively inexpensive and well worth considering to remove meatal wax.

- *Picture discrimination cards*: the authors use the Leeds Picture Discrimination Cards, which are phoneme-matched pictures (Fig. 1.4).

NOSE

- An *otoscope* can be used with a large speculum. The patient should not breathe through the nose during this brief examination or else the lens will steam up.

- *Cosmetic mirror* will show nasal patency by virtue of steaming up when held under the nose; this is especially useful in assessing very young children and babies.

- *Silver nitrate sticks* (Fig. 1.5) are useful in dealing with septal varicose vessels that are causing epistaxes. This is a straightforward procedure, which is covered in Chapter 14.

THROAT

- *Wooden tongue depressors* are abundant in the surgery.

- A *powerful pencil torch* is recommended for examination of the oral cavity and oropharynx.

Those colleagues who have had formal ENT training will be adept at using a head mirror and incident light to free both hands for instrumentation. An office desk lamp with a 100 watt bulb will suffice.

Disposable gloves will be needed for palpation of floor of mouth and buccal sulci.

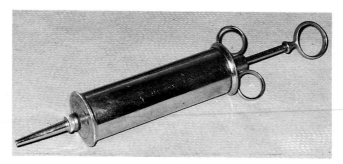

Fig. 1.2 Classic metal design ear syringe.

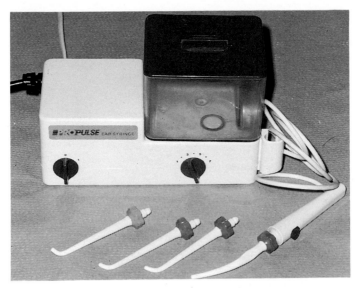

Fig. 1.3 Modern automatically pressured pump for ear syringing.

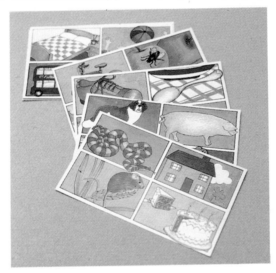

Fig. 1.4 Leeds Picture Discrimination Cards designed by Dr Mabel Yates.

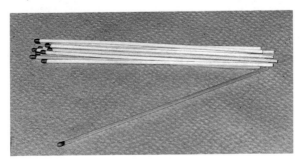

Fig. 1.5 Silver nitrate cautery sticks.

2. Equipment: application

An ENT examination requires good technique which is easy in the cooperative adult but not in a baby or anxious young child. Assistance will be needed from either a sensible parent or sympathetic member of staff in the surgery; this is portrayed in Figures 2.1 and 2.2, without labouring the point any further in the text.

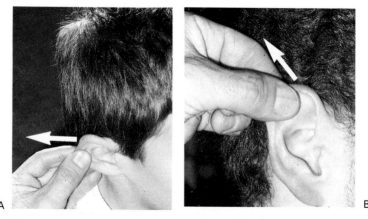

A   B

Fig. 2.1 **A** A child's ear should be retracted gently posteriorly prior to inserting the auriscope. **B** An adult's ear should be retracted postero-superiorly prior to inserting the auriscope.

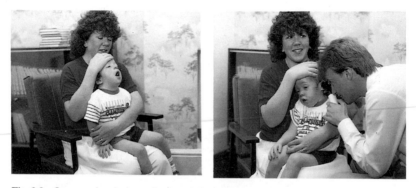

Fig. 2.2 Suggested techniques for examining the mouth and ears in a young child.

Further elaboration and illustration can be found in the appropriate chapters.

EARS

Key points:

- Presence of scars (Fig. 2.3)
- Deformity of pinna
- Appearance of external auditory canals
- Appearance of tympanic membranes (Fig. 2.4)

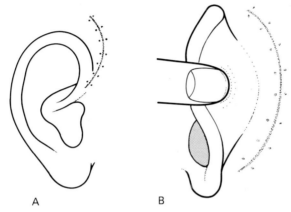

A   B

Fig. 2.3   A Scar of an endaural incision.
B Scar of a post-aural incision, seen by retracting the pinna forward.

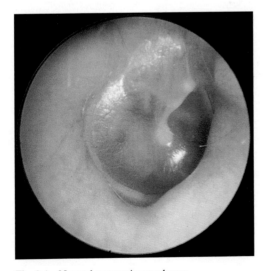

Fig. 2.4   Normal tympanic membrane.

NOSE

Key points:

- Linearity
- Patency of each nostril (Fig. 2.5)
- Little's area; i.e. that area of the septum visible on tilting the nasal tip upwards
- Vestibules
- Septum
- Turbinates (inferior turbinates are the most visible)

MOUTH, THROAT AND NECK

Key points:

- Scars or swellings
- Facial and lip symmetry
- Quality of speech
- Teeth
- Hard palate
- Tongue appearance and movement
- Buccal mucosa including retromolar trigone (Fig. 2.6) (see Glossary)
- Palpation of floor of mouth and buccal sulci, palpation of neck; this should be done in an orderly manner as in Figures 2.7a–e

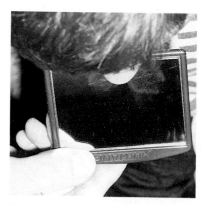

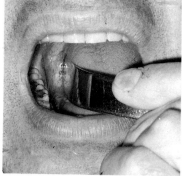

Fig. 2.5 Misting of a mirror confirms nasal patency in a young child.

Fig. 2.6 Retromolar trigone shown by tongue retraction.

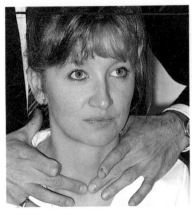

Fig. 2.7 **A** Start with the supra-sternal notch.

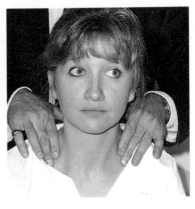

Fig. 2.7 **B** Move laterally to supraclavicular fossae.

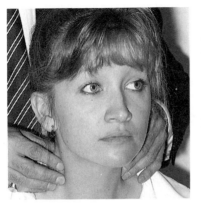

Fig. 2.7 **C** Check the posterior triangles.

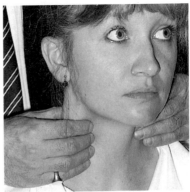

Fig. 2.7 **D** Remember to palpate around the sternomastoid muscles.

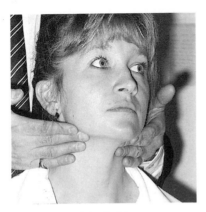

Fig. 2.7 **E** Finish off with submandibular areas.

3. Earache

- Earache is a common presenting symptom in general practice; it is often indicative of an ear infection although if the ears are both normal, a referred cause should be sought.

- Glue ear may cause an acute otitis media or vice versa.

- Rigid classification of presenting problems and differential diagnosis is difficult but the following tabulation is suggested as a useful guide based purely on the clinical experience of the authors:

When considering ear infections the possible findings are listed below but these must be considered in conjunction with history.

FINDINGS ON OTOSCOPY

Viral otitis media

- Handle of malleus flush (Fig. 3.1A).

- Bubbles sometimes seen behind membrane in conjunction with above findings (Fig. 3.1B).

- Dull tympanic membrane, i.e. diminished or no light-reflex (Fig. 3.1C).

- Peripheral vessels (Fig. 3.1E).

Bacterial otitis media

- Red and bulging (Fig. 3.1D).

- Haemorrhagic areas on membrane.

- Central perforation associated with pulsatile discharge of pus.

NB Causative features, e.g. coryza, tonsillitis, should be sought.

POINTS OF HISTORY

Viral otitis media

- Secondary to URTI or exanthemata.

- Recent onset (< 36 h).

- Mild pyrexia.

- One or both ears.

- May present in conjunction with diarrhoea and vomiting in younger children.

Bacterial otitis media

- May follow viral otitis media.

- May be a complications of tonsillitis.

- Marked pyrexia.

- More often unilateral.

- Infrequent vomiting may be a secondary feature.

- Overall deafness if both ears affected.

- Discharge of liquid wax.

- Purulent and bloody discharge from a spontaneous perforation associated with pain relief.

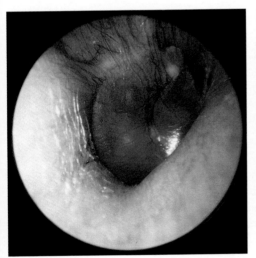

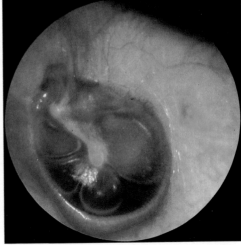

Fig. 3.1 A Malleus flush.

Fig. 3.1 B Bubbles behind the tympanic membrane in this ear were due to otitic barotrauma, but similar findings can also be seen in secretory otitis media.

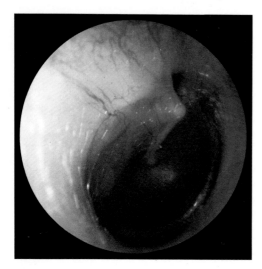

Fig. 3.1   C Dull tympanic membrane.

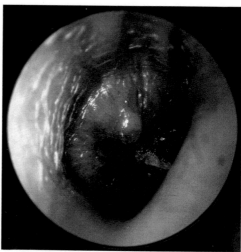

Fig. 3.1   D Bulging tympanic membrane.

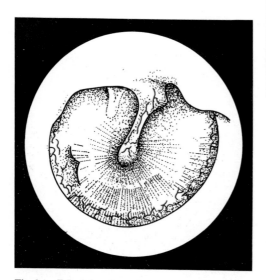

Fig. 3.1   E Peripheral vessels.

MANAGEMENT OF EARACHE

Initial presentation is within a few hours of onset of earache; this is often reported during out-of-hours emergency cover.

- Instruct on the use of paracetamol for the next 24 h because pain is the most severe symptom. The rationale for witholding antibiotics at this stage is that immunoglobulins within the exudate in the middle ear may well cope alone with the infection.

- Ensure parent understands rationale that viral otitis media is often self-limiting and that antibiotics are not necessary at this stage.

- If earache persists for more than 24 h, further GP review is necessary to treat a likely bacterial otitis media with appropriate antibiotics, e.g. cefuroxime axetil (Zinnat), cefaclor (Distaclor), ampicillin clavulinate (Augmentin). (Possibility of ampicillin-resistant haemophilus should be remembered.)

- Review in two weeks to exclude secretory otitis media (syn glue ear) (Fig. 3.2) which may occur secondarily to both viral and bacterial otitis media.

- Secretory otitis causing persistent deafness (see Ch. 5)
- Recurrent acute otitis media causing parental or GP concern REFER
- Earache complicated by ear discharge REFER
- Earache with history of underlying ear disease needs investigation REFER
- If tympanic membrane looks normal. See 'Other Local Causes'.

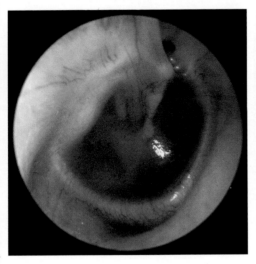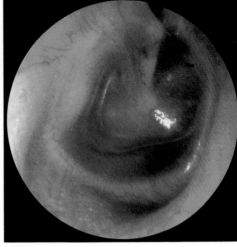

B

Fig. 3.2   Secretory otitis media **A** Honey-coloured tympanic membrane. **B** Air-fluid meniscus.

Sequelae of viral and bacterial otitis media

- Complete resolution – no further action.

- Recurrence of earache – see above.

- Secretory otitis media
    — asymptomatic – observe
    — deafness – see Ch. 5
    — recurrent – REFER .

- Acute perforation (Fig. 3.3) may heal spontaneously – advise against water and shampoos in ear. Observe and review in one month to ensure complete resolution.

- Chalk patches (syn tympanosclerosis) (Fig. 3.4) is a long-term sequel to infection – no action.

- Chronic perforation – see Ch. 10.

Acute otitis media de novo is less common in adults than in childhood and a history of previous ear disease should be sought.

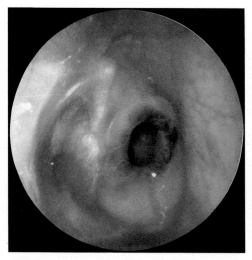 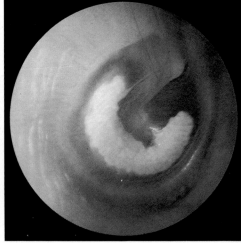

Fig. 3.3   Acute otitis media resulting in a temporary perforation.

Fig. 3.4   Tympanosclerosis.

OTHER LOCAL CAUSES

Otitis externa

Primary otitis externa represents eczema and secondary infection of skin in the external auditory canal and meatal orifice, sometimes involving the pinna. It is usually bilateral and includes the following features:

- Itch or ache
- Discharge, usually watery
- Slight deafness or fullness
- Aching down the neck from associated external jugular glands

Management

- If very mild with minimal debris, use trial of antibiotic/steroid mixture drops, three times a day for 5 days, e.g. gentamycin hydrocortisone (Gentisone HC) compound. **Avoid contamination with shampoos, etc.**

- If facilities available, broad spectrum antibiotic cream on ½ inch ribbon gauze, three times a week (Fig. 3.5); if not REFER.

- If condition fails to settle REFER for microsuction (see Chapter 4).

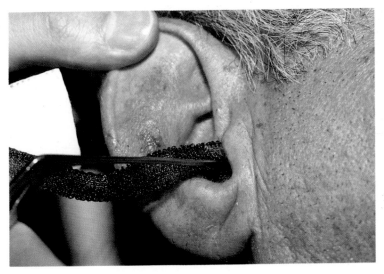

Fig. 3.5 Ear packed with a ½-inch ribbon gauze. The above example shows a glycerine and ichthammol wick, but where there is a reasonably wide lumen an antibiotic cream can be used.

Pitfalls

Unilateral otitis externa may be:

- Traumatic in origin
- Secondary to a perforation. If perforation is not obvious REFER for microsuction and examination
- Pseudomonal otitis externa

Furuncle

- A boil in external auditory meatus of one ear (Fig. 3.6)
- Very painful
- Diagnosed by pulling upwards and backwards; the pain is made worse during this manoeuvre

Treatment

- Glycerin and ichthammol on ½ inch ribbon gauze (see Fig. 3.5).

- Analgesics by mouth although if patient debilitated by pain and loss of sleep, REFER acutely for in-patient management.

LESS COMMON LOCAL CAUSES OF EARACHE

- Herpes zoster oticus and facial palsy (Fig. 3.7) REFER
- Bullous haemorrhagic myringitis (Fig. 3.8)
    — earache
    — red bullae on membrane
    — treat with analgesics. If acute otitis media supervenes, oral antibiotics may prove necessary

- Perichondritis; REFER acutely for in-patient management

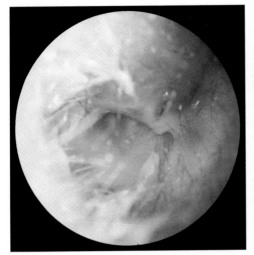

Fig. 3.6   Furuncle in external auditory canal.

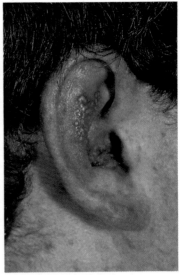

Fig. 3.7   Herpes zoster vesicles on the concha.

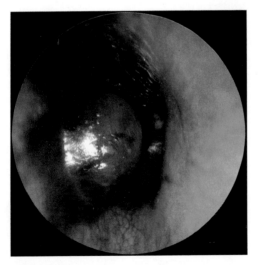

Fig. 3.8   Bullous haemorrhagic myringitis.

CAUSES OF REFERRED EARACHE

- Tonsillitis
- Glandular fever
    - treat with simple analgesics and bedrest
    - if severe, REFER acutely for in-patient management

- Temporo-mandibular joint dysfunction (Fig. 3.9) occurs from malocclusion of teeth, aggravated by grinding of teeth during sleep and associated earache without pyrexia. This may interrupt sleep; dental REFERRAL for assessment and night splint
- Cervical arthritis
- Tumours in mouth, throat or sinuses with their associated symptoms and signs
- Unerupted or impacted wisdom teeth, dental REFERRAL

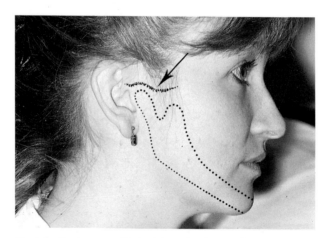

Fig. 3.9   Temperomandibular joint pain often presents as earache.

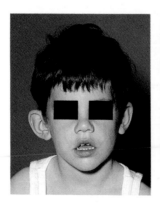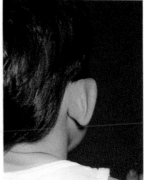

Fig. 3.10   Displacement of the pinna is a feature of acute mastoiditis.

Pitfalls

- Any unwell infant should have the ears examined to exclude acute otitis media.

- Severity of parental distress does not necessarily reflect severity of disease.

- In the management of otitis media, a 24 h treatment just with analgesics without antibiotics is not detrimental to the outcome.

- Any recurrent purulent disease of middle or internal ear, exclude diabetes.

- Adult secretory otitis media de novo needs REFERRAL to exclude obstructive lesion of nasopharynx, e.g. carcinoma.

- Mastoid abscess must not be diagnosed in the presence of a normal of near normal tympanic membrane.

- Mastoiditis (Fig. 3.10) is part of the inflammatory process of the middle ear cleft (otitis media) and this will settle with the appropriate conservative treatment. Only when this becomes complicated into a mastoid abscess should this be REFERRED .

- It is a common mistake to diagnose minimal tenderness over the mastoid tip as requiring acute surgical intervention in the presence of a middle ear cleft infection (otitis media).

- Mastoid abscess occurs behind or above the ear and may coexist with a cholesteatoma. There is marked local and constitutional disturbance REFER .

4. Ear discharge

If there is a history of previous ear surgery on the discharging ear or evidence of any surgical scarring around the ear, a detailed examination will be required REFER.

The above group excluded, ear discharge can occur from the following.

OTITIS EXTERNA

This is an eczematous condition of the external auditory canals ± pinna causing itch, pain and moisture (Fig. 4.1). It usually occurs bilaterally; unilateral cases are usually secondary to:

- Middle ear disease
- Trauma, e.g. hearing aid friction
- Furuncle
- Pseudomonas otitis externa (usually in diabetics)
- Malignancy very rarely

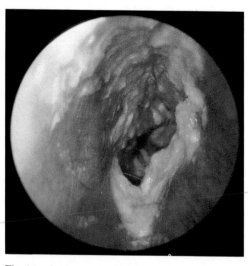

Fig. 4.1 Otitis externa, gross.

Points of history in otitis externa:

- Previous history of otitis externa, because it is often recurrent.

- Itch is predominant although pain can be associated, occasionally severe.

- Sensation of fullness because of debris accumulation.

- Discharge is usually *not* foul-smelling.

- Mild hearing loss may occur because of debris and swelling.

MIDDLE EAR DISEASE

This must be discharging through a perforation of the tympanic membrane.

TRAUMA OR FOREIGN BODY

REFER SOON

MANAGEMENT OF EAR DISCHARGE

Absolute indications for REFERRAL are:

- Ipselateral facial palsy or other cranial nerve disorders
- True vertigo suggesting cholesteatoma
- Foul-smelling discharge suggesting cholesteatoma
- CSF otorrhoea following a head injury
- Previous ipselateral ear surgery

Treatment on the practice premises

- Initial treatment is with topical antibiotic/steroid compound drops for 5 days.

- If the patient is diabetic, a swab should be sent off to exclude pseudomonas; if so REFER as this particular condition can be severely erosive.

- Advise on avoidance of shampoos, conditioners, swimming, bath water and saunas (because of excess sweat).

- If the above fails, repeat otoscopy which may show:

(1)   Narrow canals with swollen walls (Fig. 4.2)

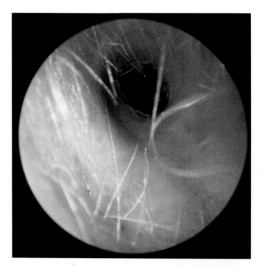

Fig. 4.2   External canal stenosis because of swollen walls.

- Treat with glycerin and ichthammol ribbon gauze (Fig. 4.3)

½ inch wide

2 inches long

three times a week for 2 weeks inserted by practice nurse (appropriately trained by local ENT department)

resolution

canal still swollen REFER

canal open but debris still present; for further advice follow (2)

(2) Excessive debris

treat with ½ inch ribbon
gauze in situ for 5 days with
antibiotic installation onto
gauze 3 times a day, e.g.
Trimovate ointment,
Vioform HC

resolution

debris removed leaving
inflamed wall, use drops for
further 5 days without gauze.
If this does not settle
REFER

persistent debris REFER
for microscopic suction

- Any associated earache should be treated with analgesics.

- Any associated external jugular lymph node swelling or discomfort, additional treatment with oral antibiotics for 5 days is recommended.

- For itch that does not quickly respond to dressing as outlined above, an antihistamine may be useful, e.g. terfenadine (Triludan), astemizole (Hismanal), cetirizine (Zirtek).

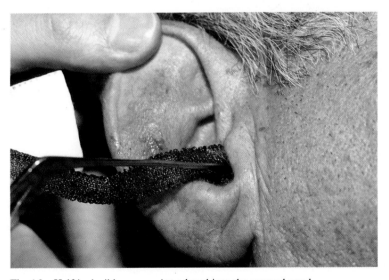

Fig. 4.3 Half-inch ribbon gauze introduced into the external canal.

FURTHER EVALUATION

- When ear dries up, a tympanic perforation may be visible and should be looked for in a unilateral otitis externa.

- Perforations occur
    - centrally (Fig. 4.4**A**); review for six weeks. If not healed, see Chapter 10
    - in attic (Fig. 4.4**B**) REFER

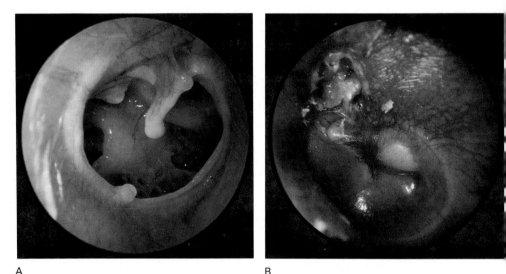

A   B

Fig. 4.4   **A** A total perforation in this case represents an extension of a large central perforation. **B** Attic perforation of the left tympanic membrane (at 11 o'clock position).

PITFALLS

- Any unilateral otitis externa should have a tympanic perforation excluded. As mentioned before, a foul-smelling discharge is indicative of cholesteatoma and patient should therefore be REFERRED .

- Opportunistic infection by fungus (Fig. 4.5**A** and **B**), commonly candida species and *Aspergillus niger*, may have occurred because of:
    - overuse of topical antibiotic drops, steroid drops or compound preparations
    - diabetes
    - general immunosuppression.

- Routine swabs from ears are unnecessary unless patient is diabetic where pseudomonal otitis externa is more likely.

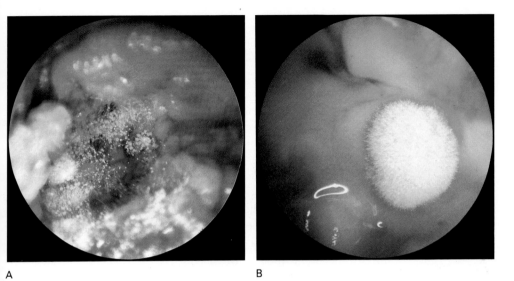

A

B

Fig. 4.5 **A** Spores diagnostic of a fungal infection. **B** Fungal hyphae.

5. Childhood deafness

If a parent suspects that their child is deaf, the child should be considered deaf until otherwise proven. Overall deafness implicates bilateral hearing loss; it is unlikely that a unilateral childhood deafness presents as an overall inability to hear.

A useful way of managing these children is to consider whether or not there is associated earache.

WITH EARACHE

Consider:

- Acute otitis media (Fig. 5.1)
- May be directly preceded by an upper respiratory tract infection

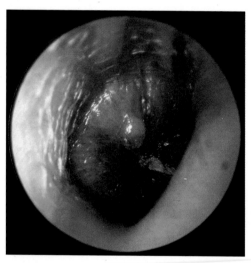

Fig. 5.1 Acute otitis media with characteristic bulging tympanic membranes.

WITHOUT EARACHE

Consider:

- Hard impacted wax; soft wax is unlikely to cause deafness.

- Bilateral secretory otitis media is a likely cause; this may occur with or without a preceding upper respiratory tract infection.

- History of pre-, peri- or post-natal complications affecting the sensori-neural component should be sought.

- History of meningitis or severe exanthemata should be sought but the diagnosis of deafness may well have been picked up at that time.

- History of head injury with concussion.

- Congenital malformation of the hearing apparatus may well be associated with pinna deformity; this is usually noticed at neonatal examination.

MANAGEMENT OF PAINFUL DEAFNESS

- As acute otitis earache (see Ch. 3); 24 h of a paediatric paracetamol preparation in appropriate maximum doses.

- Beyond 24 h; a 3-day course of an appropriate maximum dose of an antibiotic for the patient's age.

- A spontaneous discharge from affected ear will relieve pain but a secretory otitis media (syn glue ear) may supervene and the cycle restarted once the acute perforation has healed.

- If earache settles but deafness persists, treat as deafness without earache.

- Nose drops do not contribute.

MANAGEMENT OF PAINLESS DEAFNESS

- It is important to gain the history from the parent as to what has been noticed to arouse their suspicions of deafness in the child.

- Assess for speech and reading ability; if delayed REFER for full audiological and developmental assessment.

Examination of the ear and the tympanic membrane may show:

(1)   Wax and debris

Wax may be syringed provided a perforation of the tympanic membrane is not suspected (Fig. 5.2). Unless the wax is hard and the plug large, syringing will not cure the deafness but merely allow otoscopic examination of the membrane; if wax is very hard, use 5% sodium bicarbonate drops three times a day for 5 days before further syringing.

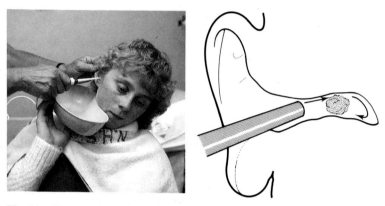

Fig. 5.2   When syringing wax, the stream of water must be directed along the roof of the external canal to avoid traumatic rupture of the tympanic membrane.

(2)   Glue ear

This is the most likely finding, diagnosed by:

- Visible blood vessels on the tympanic membrane which are often present peripherally and radially (Fig. 5.3A).
- Honey-coloured tympanic membrane (Fig. 5.3B).
- Absence of light-reflex.
- Blue discolouration of tympanic membrane (Fig. 5.3C).
- Presence of fluid levels (Fig. 5.3D) or air bubbles (Fig. 5.3E) behind the tympanic membrane. Handle of malleus in a horizontal position.
- Split light-reflex which indicates a retraction of the tympanic membrane. This is often found in glue ear, but can also be associated with other causes of mild tympanic membrane retraction without glue (Fig. 5.3F).

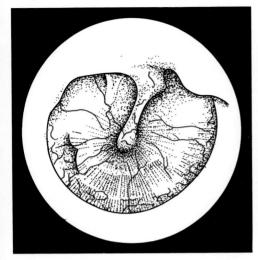

Fig. 5.3   A Radial blood vessels.

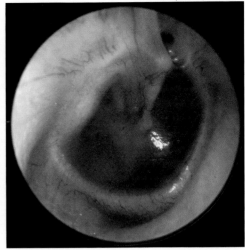

Fig. 5.3   B Honey-coloured tympanic membrane.

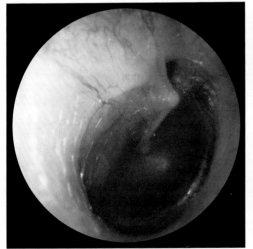

Fig. 5.3   C Air-fluid meniscus.

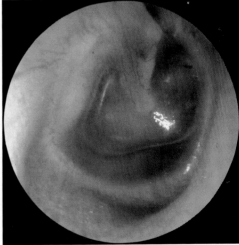

Fig. 5.3   D Dull tympanic membrane.

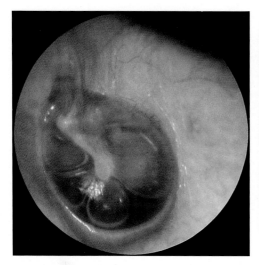

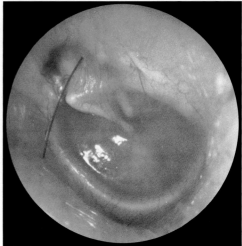

Fig. 5.3 E Bubbles behind the tympanic membrane in this ear were due to otitic barotrauma, but similar findings can also be seen in secretory otitis media.

Fig. 5.3 F Retracted tympanic membrane showing a split light reflex and a horizontal tilt to the handle of malleus.

When managing secretory otitis media (syn glue ear), consider:

- Acute otitis media and secretory otitis media may lead to one another.

- Assessment of speech and reading development; if delayed REFER as this indicates prolonged glue ear; spontaneous resolution in the near future is unlikely.

- If there is no developmental delay, observe at 2-monthly intervals to assess parental, nursery or school report of any change in hearing.

- Failure to show any improvement after the first 2 months of assessment REFER.

- With intermittent fluctuation of hearing, continue to observe at two-monthly intervals.

- The older the child towards the age of 10, the greater the likelihood of spontaneous resolution.

- Nasal drops, oral decongestants, mucolytics and antibiotics are unlikely to help.

(3) Tympanic perforation – REFER

Assessment of a child's hearing can often be performed within the surgery using Leeds Picture Discrimination Cards (see Fig. 1.4) and whispered voice at 3 feet (Fig. 5.4).

- Age 0–3: refer to health visitor who will liaise.
- Age 3–6: picture discrimination cards.
- Age   6: whispered voice test using easy numbers.

Pure-tone audiometry can be arranged through the health visitor **but** the whispered voice test is more valuable because it tests not only threshold but discrimination between different sounds.

PITFALLS

- If parent or guardian feels their child is deaf and the ears and membranes are both normal, suspect underlying sensori-neural deafness. REFER
- In a child deaf with secretory otitis media, do remember that a sensori-neural deafness may also be present. This should be borne in mind especially with a markedly deaf child. REFER

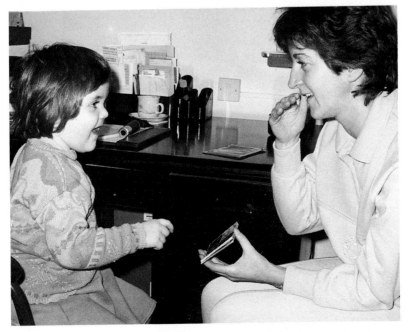

Fig. 5.4 When using the Leeds Picture Discrimination Cards, the tester should use a whispered voice with the lips obscured at approximately 3 feet from the child.

6. Adult deafness

This is normally of slow onset and the patient will have socially inadequate hearing with bilateral deafness; unilateral hearing loss causes a more specific deafness, for example, the telephone or direction of voice at a business meeting.

POINTS OF HISTORY

- Previous ear surgery.

- Childhood illness (exanthemata) sometimes involves a sensori-neural loss, as well as a conductive loss.

- Head injury or direct ear injury.

- Severe systemic illness and ototoxic drugs.

- Occupational history may give a story of prolonged noise exposure.

- Hobbies, such as rifle shooting (usually over many years) may suggest this as a contributory cause.

- Family history of deafness suggests otosclerosis or familial sensori-neural deafness.

FINDINGS THAT CAN BE MANAGED IN THE SURGERY

- Wax; in the absence of a history of perforation or previous ear operation, 5% sodium bicarbonate drops can be administered for 5 days, followed by syringing. (OTC drops may well cause a chemical otitis externa.)

TESTING THE HEARING IN THE SURGERY

- Whispered voice; assessment at three feet distance by masking the contralateral ear (Fig. 6.1).

- Conversational voice at three feet distance from each ear with gentle tragal rubbing of untested ear to prevent crossover of sound.

- General conversational voice with lips obscured from patient's view.

- Tuning fork tests are quite helpful, although wide variation makes really accurate diagnosis impossible.

  — Weber and Rinné tests (Fig. 6.2, see over) to distinguish between conductive deafness and sensori-neural deafness. A 512-Hz tuning fork is recommended; higher frequencies fade too frequently and lower frequencies cause excessive vibration.

- An interrupted pure-tone audiogram, useful if available (see Chapter 7).

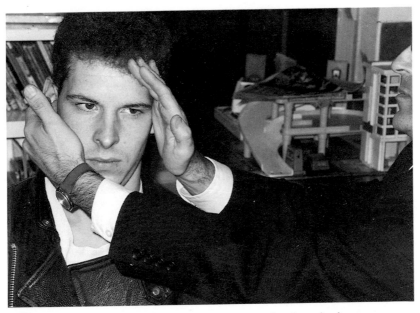

Fig. 6.1 When performing a whispered voice test, ensure that the patient's eyes are shielded to prevent lipreading. The opposite tragus is lightly rubbed to prevent the sound being heard by the other ear.

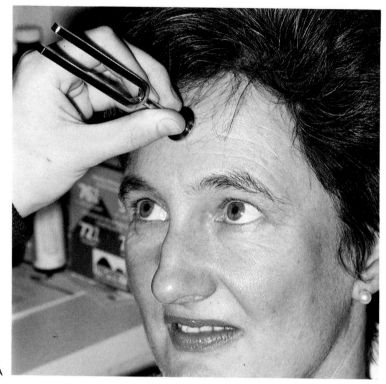

A

Fig. 6.2 A Weber test. A tuning fork placed on the forehead should be heard equally in both ears. If the sound is heard better in one ear, either (i) that ear may have a conductive deafness or (ii) the other ear has a sensorineural (nerve) deafness.

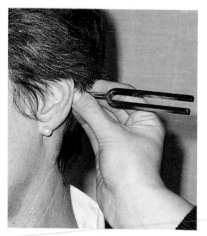

B

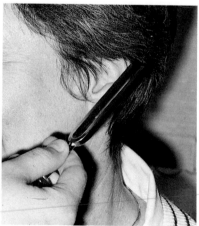

C

Fig. 6.2 B Rinné test. The tuning fork is placed on the mastoid process behind the ear. The patient indicates when the sound is no longer heard. **C** The fork is then held adjacent to the ear. The fork can still be heard when that ear is normal, or when the ear has a sensorineural deafness. In a conductive loss the sound is heard better behind the ear than adjacent to it.

WHEN TO REFER

- If wax removal fails to improve reduced hearing which is confirmed on testing.

- All sudden deafness should be REFERRED if wax is not visible.

PITFALLS

- Even if malingering is suspected in relation to an industrial or criminal claim, this should be REFERRED for audiological testing.

7. Pure tone audiometry – nature and interpretation

A pure tone audiogram (PTA) is a chart showing hearing levels (measured in decibels) at various frequencies (measured in cycles per second or Herz).

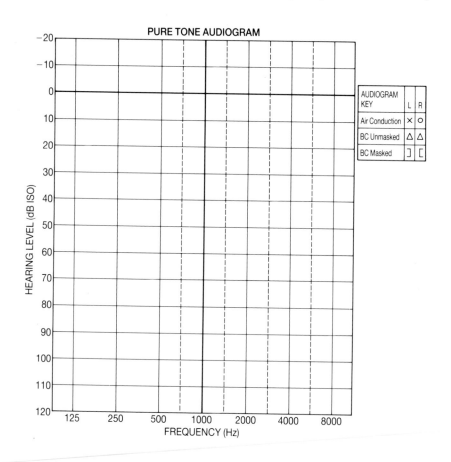

The vertical scale of decibels is logarithmic; that is to say, if two sounds differ by 20 decibels, the difference between them in intensity will be 10^2 or 100-fold. Likewise if the difference between those two sounds is 30 decibels, the difference in intensity will be 10^3 or 1000-fold, etc.

The audiographic scales are based on a population average: hence −10 decibels means better than the population average of 0 decibels.

Each frequency is specifically tested for:

- Air conduction via ear phones. This measures sound levels heard via the normal processes, i.e. a sound wave which hits the tympanic membrane which is then transmitted via the ossicles to the inner ear and the electrical pathways systems, i.e. cochlea and auditory nerve.

- Bone conduction via a transducer applied to the mastoid bone. (A masking noise has to be applied to the ear which is not being tested.) This reflects the ability of the electrical systems of the ear to sense and transduce sound, i.e. the function of the cochlea and auditory nerve.

Hearing problems can be divided into two categories:

- Conductive loss
- Sensori-neural (nerve) loss

CONDUCTIVE LOSS

This represents a loss of sound in the conduction system of the ear between the drum and cochlea (via the ossicles). Reduction of hearing can then occur with:

- Glue ear
- Large perforations
- Dislocation, destruction or adhesion of the ossicles

The audiogram shows a normal sensori-neural (nerve) pattern, but a reduced conductive hearing pattern as below:

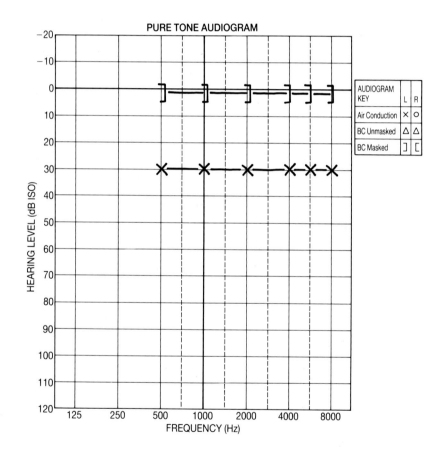

SENSORI-NEURAL LOSS

This represents a defect within the electrical aspect of the ear, i.e. the cochlea and auditory nerve. The audiogram shows reduced levels for both air conduction and bone conduction.

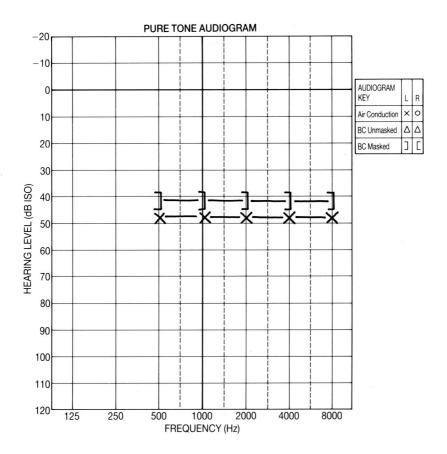

Presbycusis

Hearing loss with age is a variant of a sensori-neural hearing loss, but mainly occurs at high frequencies.

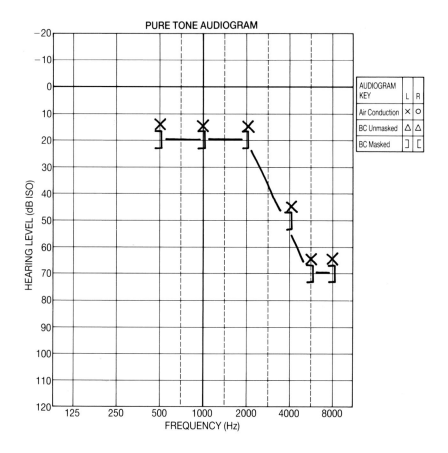

Sensori-neural hearing loss normally requires referral to an ENT out-patients' department for assessment. REFER

Mixed losses are also commonly found, e.g. presbycusis on top of long-standing middle ear disease such as tympanosclerotic scarring.

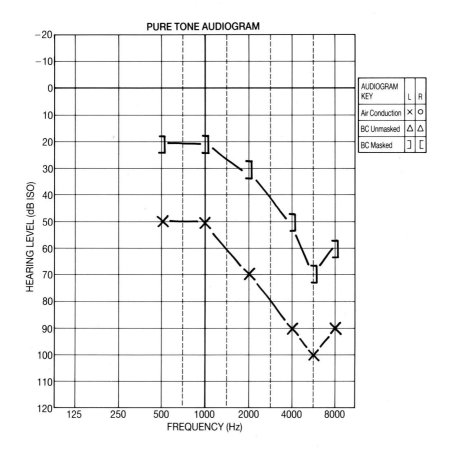

8. Services for patients with impaired hearing

Once diagnosed as having a hearing problem, a child is referred to a teacher for the deaf. This department helps plan educational development, auditory training and arrange for the fitting of a hearing aid if appropriate. There is a close communication between:

- Parents
- Local ENT department
- Local audiology clinic
- Primary health care team

The child's education is planned from an early age as soon as the chronic deafness is diagnosed. Hopefully they will be able to achieve competence in language by the age of five.

EDUCATION

- *Normal schools* are attended by 50% of children who have irreversible deafness and are visited by teachers of the deaf. These teachers help and advise on:
  - use of hearing aids
  - help with lip reading
  - assessment of the child's progress
- *Special units* are situated in some schools and, indeed, this is now the favoured trend away from schools for the deaf. These units offer:
  - induction loop aids which amplify the teacher's voice. This in turn is picked up by the child's hearing aid
  - radio-hearing aids, which comprise a radio-microphone hand-held by the teacher. The radio-microphone transmits to a radio-receiver worn by the child.
- *Schools for the deaf* are still part of the education system, although the trend is towards special units within normal schools.
- *Additional skills* include manual communication known as 'signing'. These manual skills are combined with oral communication to form 'total communication'.

DOMESTIC DEVICES

These improve communication for the deaf, and include modifications to:

- Telephones

  (a) Bell — extension bells
  — flashing lights
  — amplified bells, buzzers and hooters
  (b) Handset — amplification
  — adjustable volume control
  — induction couplers within the handset will amplify sound in the hearing aid when it is set in the 'T' position (Fig. 8.1)

- Television
  — separate loudspeakers
  — induction loops which generate an electromagnetic field; this in turn generates a current and signal in the hearing aid when set in the 'T' position. This facility is available in some cinemas and auditoria
  — Ceefax and Oracle offering subtitles and specific services for the deaf

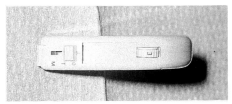

Fig. 8.1 Hearing aids have an OTM switch. O is off, M is the normal operating position and T is used in combination with induction loop mechanisms. The volume control is numbered 1 to 4.

USEFUL ADDRESSES

- Royal National Institute for the Deaf
  106 Gower Street
  London WC1E 6AH
  Tel: 071 387–8033

- City Lit Centre for Deaf People & Speech Therapy (adults)
  Keeley House
  Keeley Street
  London WC2B 4BA
  Tel: 071 430–0548

- Link
  British Centre for Deafened People
  19 Hartfield Road
  Eastbourne
  East Sussex BR21 2AR
  (This organization is particularly useful for the suddenly deafened.)

9. Tinnitus

Tinnitus is a descriptive term applied to noises, either in the ear or head. Patients will often describe the noise as a whistling kettle although some will describe a pulsatile quality synchronous with the heartbeat.

Tinnitus can be considered as subjective or objective.

SUBJECTIVE TINNITUS

This is often secondary to sensori-neural auditory defects. It can be exacerbated by middle ear disease which prevents ambient masking sound from reaching the inner ear.

Many adult patients are extremely anxious about their *subjective* tinnitus, in case it represents sinister disease, such as brain tumour; appropriate reassurance will be required. Anxiety itself will accentuate the tinnitus.

Most patients with subjective tinnitus will give a history of **deafness**:

- If the deafness is socially embarrassing, REFER for audiology and aiding, which may well quell the tinnitus as well as relieve deafness.

- If mild, reassurance that the tinnitus represents the ravages of wear and tear on the inner ear. This reassurance may well reduce the element of anxiety with consequent reduction in tinnitus.

If tinnitus is severely affecting the patient, REFER for tinnitus masker, which is effective when hearing is reasonable.

- Patients with tympanic abnormalities should be referred for thorough assessment.

- Children occasionally complain of *subjective* tinnitus; secretory otitis media is often the cause (see Chapter 5).

OBJECTIVE TINNITUS

This is when the noise is actually heard by other people standing nearby. This is very rare and should be ‖REFERRED‖.

It should be noted that there is no virtue whatever in prescribing oral medication for tinnitus per se although secondary problems such as sleeplessness or depression will need specific treatment.

Those patients who are disabled by tinnitus may well benefit by writing to:

> The Tinnitus Association
> Royal National Institution of the Deaf
> 105 Gower Street
> London   WC1E 6AH

This organization distributes high-quality periodicals which keep patients up to date with tinnitus research and boost their morale.

10. Tympanic perforations

Tympanic membrane perforations can be managed in general practice by considering whether they are:

- Attic perforations (Fig. 10.1A)
- Central perforations (Fig. 10.1B)

ATTIC PERFORATIONS

These are diagnosed by:

- Otoscopic detection of a superiorly placed small perforation ± granulation tissue ± visible cholesteatoma.

- Inference, i.e. a foul-smelling discharge and debris which obscures a clear view of the tympanic membrane.

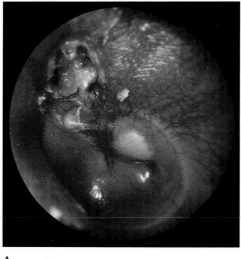
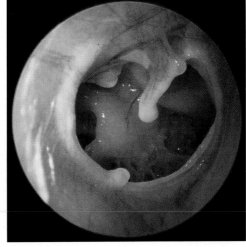

A   B

Fig. 10.1 **A** Attic perforation of the left tympanic membrane (at 11 o'clock position). **B** A total perforation in this case represents an extension of a large central perforation.

The presenting symptoms and conditions caused by cholesteatoma (Fig. 10.2) are:

- deafness
- foul otorrhoea
- earache
- ipsilateral facial palsy
- vertigo
- abscess over mastoid bone
- meningitis

Management

- All suspected attic perforations or cholesteatoma should be REFERRED for microscopy and possible surgery.

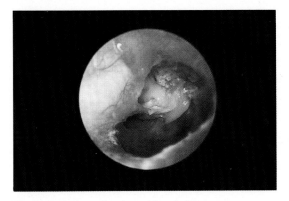

Fig. 10.2   Attic perforation with a cholesteatoma.

CENTRAL PERFORATIONS

- Can be safely observed for a period by the GP.

- Occurring in response to trauma or otitis media may well heal spontaneously.

Management

- If the tympanic membrane is obscured by discharge, then prescribe a 5-day course of antibiotic ear drops (cf Chapter 4).

- When the perforation is dry, then observe and advise the patient to prevent water entering the ear by the use of 'Blue-Tac®' or cottonwool smeared with Vaseline®. Review the patient in 6 weeks; thereafter, the patient should report back with any further trouble.

INDICATIONS FOR REFERRAL

- Recurrent otorrhoea
- Earache from secondary otitis externa
- Deafness
- Troublesome vertigo due to the caloric effect of cold air
- Occupational necessity for intact tympanic membranes, e.g. armed forces, hobbies, etc.

Should a symptomless perforation persist, the GP can confidently reassure the patient that no active treatment is required, except keeping the ear from bath and swimming-pool water, etc.

PITFALLS

- If a perforation occurs as a result of criminal assault, it would be as well to obtain an audiogram at initial presentation, as well as after 6 weeks, by which time spontaneous healing will have taken place.

11. Dizziness, giddiness and vertigo

- These are the patient's words to describe his predicament. The GP assesses the history to ascertain whether the symptoms are of true vertigo.

- Vertigo is specifically a hallucination of rotatory movement. The history from the patient must indicate a definite sensation of spinning.

- If the history does not include spinning, the symptom is not vertigo, more of light-headedness, which requires a general medical assessment.

- If the symptom of vertigo is convincing, then the general practitioner has to assess whether the origin is:
  — otogenic; or
  — CNS.

OTOGENIC

(1) Ménière's syndrome

This is all too frequently diagnosed because it is assumed to be synonymous with recurrent vertigo and deafness. Ménière's syndrome represents an idiopathic endolymphatic hydrops, where the endolymph channel of the inner ear is expanded relative to the perilymph channels. To diagnose Ménière's syndrome, the following symptoms should be present:

- Vertigo and nausea
- Change of hearing directly associated with the episodes of spinning
- Sense of fullness or blocking of the ear
- Tinnitus classically appears to change its usual pitch in relation to the episodes of spinning
- Clustering of attacks

Management

REFER for assessment and confirmation of the diagnosis as treatment may subsequently be life long. There is a great variation in modes of treatment for this condition and we suggest that each patient will require a management plan which is arrived at by communication between GP, hospital consultant and patient. Possible drug treatment includes drugs to reduce the hydrops, e.g. betahistine (Serc) or thymoxamine (Opilon) and/or labyrinthine sedatives, e.g. cinnarizine.

(2)   Viral labyrinthitis

This is suggested by the key points:

- Recent viral URTI
- Associated nausea or vomiting
- No associated loss of hearing necessarily
- Normal tympanic membrane
- History will start with true vertigo and will usually modify into a sense of general imbalance before complete resolution

Management

- Reassurance that it is self-limiting in a few weeks, occasionally months
- Advise patient to remain in bed if necessary
- Normal activities to be curtailed
- Labyrinthine sedatives; if vomiting precludes oral route, use suppositories, parenteral administration or buccal preparation, i.e. Buccastem
- If persistent over 6 weeks REFER

(3)   Benign positional vertigo

This is suggested by the key points:

- Fleeting vertigo usually when the patient lies down with head in a triggering position (usually one particular ear towards pillow).

- Vertigo can be elicited in the surgery by lying patient on a couch with head (supported by clinician's hand) over the top edge, with one ear lowermost. The patient is instructed to sit up quickly and fix stare ahead; nystagmus associated with resulting vertigo may be seen for a few seconds. The process is reversed again, to elicit nystagmus.

- Normal or 'non-acute' tympanic membranes.

Management

- Reassurance.

- Advise patient to remain in the triggering position for as long as possible until vertigo has settled, rather than 'escape'. This will improve central compensation.

- Labyrinthine sedatives may not be wholly successful but are worth a try.

- If persistent beyond 3 months ⏍REFER⏍.

CNS ORIGIN

(1)   Vertebro-basilar insufficiency

This is suggested by the key points:

- Association with neck extension and rotation
- Normal tympanic membranes
- Associated neck pain related to underlying cervical spondylitis
- May be generalized features of arteriosclerosis, e.g. bruits, claudication
- Occasional TIA symptoms

Management

- Cervical collar
- Reappraisal of life-style
- Specific treatment of osteoarthritis if applicable

⏍URGENT REFERRAL⏍ is necessary when vertigo is associated with:

- Attic cholesteatoma
- Ear discharge
- Deafness
- Facial palsy
- Headaches and neurological abnormalities, e.g. PICA (posterior inferior cerebellar artery) syndrome, incipient hydrocephalus
- Previous ear surgery
- Recent head injury

Following ENT specialist investigation and treatment, there are a number of patients with conditions manageable thereafter by the general practitioner:

- Ménière's syndrome
- Vertebro-basilar insufficiency
- Neurological conditions
- Financially-motivated compensation-associated conditions

FISTULA TEST

In cases of attic cholesteatoma with or without ear discharge, it is quite possible for the lateral semicircular canal to be eroded. In such cases of cholesteatoma and a history of vertigo, the fistula test may well confirm this scenario but not always. The method is simple; the clinician presses the external meatus of the affected ear by pressing the tragus. The patient will immediately have vertigo and the eyes will turn away to the good side; when the finger pressure is removed, the eyes will return to the centre followed by a little nystagmus.

PITFALLS

- Patients with loss of consciousness associated with vertigo should be sent for a neurological opinion.

- Light-headedness should also be asked for specifically. Remember that both symptoms of vertigo and light-headedness may coexist and should be unravelled from the history.

- Presbycusis and presbystasis are common problems in the elderly. A history of light-headedness only will **exclude** conditions such as Ménière's syndrome. Even if there is a genuine history of vertigo from, say, vertebro-basilar insufficiency, unrelated presbycusis does not constitute Ménière's syndrome.

12. Facial palsy

This is classified into:

- Upper motor neurone. This spares the ipsilateral frontalis muscle and is commonly part of a cerebrovascular accident.

- Lower motor neurone lesion which involves the ipsilateral frontalis along with the other ipsilateral facial muscles (Fig. 12.1).

The lower motor neurone lesion will be assumed in this section. Bell's palsy is a diagnosis of exclusion once the foregoing has been ruled out.

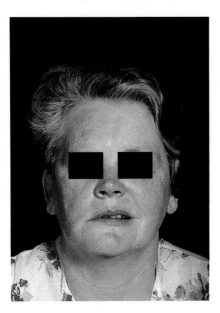

Fig. 12.1 Lower motor neurone facial palsy.

HERPES ZOSTER

Shingles affecting the ipsilateral auricular skin, palate and pharynx as well as the facial nerve. The acoustic nerve may be affected. This scenario is also known as Ramsay-Hunt syndrome (Fig. 12.2).

Management

- Analgesics
- Acyclovir (Zovirax) orally and topically
- Corneal protection (especially during sleep) using eyepad and hypromellose eye drops ('artificial tears')
- Electromyographic (EMG) assessment via local ENT colleague to help assess prognosis
- Management of patient's morale in respect of their expectations because facial recovery may not occur

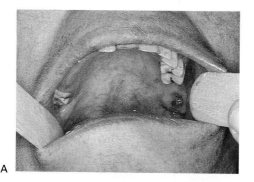

A

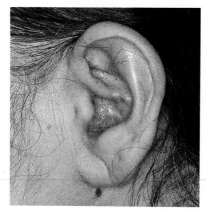

B

Fig. 12.2 A In Ramsey-Hunt syndrome Herpes zoster vesicles can be seen on the ipsilateral half of the palate. A tooth has been removed in the mistaken diagnosis of decay; in fact it was the prodromal pain in the palate and gum of Ramsay-Hunt syndrome. A palatal rash subsequently developed. **B** Herpes zoster vesicles on the concha.

ADVANCING MIDDLE EAR DISEASE

If a lower motor neurone facial palsy occurs in association with an ipsi-lateral otorrhoea or identifiable cholesteatoma REFER.

POST-TRAUMATIC CASES

These will probably present to the Accident and Emergency Department, although an occasional patient will present to the general practitioner's surgery and should be REFERRED to the ENT department forthwith.

BELL'S PALSY

This is a diagnosis of exclusion.

- 75% fully recover in 3 weeks; failure of resolution after 3 weeks should prompt REFERRAL. The likely explanation of delayed resolution is degeneration of some or all of the facial nerve fibres.

- May be preceded by pain around the ipsilateral ear.

- Patients may well present to the GP fearful that they are having a stroke.

- Taste fibres in the trigeminal nerve accompany sensory branches to the anterior two-thirds of tongue. Taste and lacrimation recover early.

- Management of patient's morale in respect of their expectations, especially if recovery does not occur quickly.

- ACTH and steroids have not proven to be beneficial.

- The eye should be protected in the early stages with artificial tear drops and eyepad, especially when the patient is outdoors or asleep.

- If secondary corneal damage is suspected, REFER to ophthalmologist.

- Slowly resolving cases should be sent for transcutaneous nerve stimulation at the local physiotherapy department, to prevent facial muscular contracture.

- Alternative neurological diagnosis should be considered in cases with multiple neuropathies.

13. Nasal blockage

This is the sensation of reduced air flow, either unilaterally or bilaterally. The basic subdivisions are:

- Mucosal swelling due to:
    - coryza
    - allergic rhinitis
    - vaso-motor rhinitis (syn non-allergic)
    - polypi

- Septal deviation either
    - of traumatic origin
    - idiopathic

- Valvular inspiratory collapse at one or both nostrils

- Nasopharyngeal obstruction from
    - enlarged adenoids
    - polypi
    - tumour

ASSOCIATED POINTS OF THE HISTORY

The differential diagnosis of mucosal swelling is often discernable by the swelling.

Allergic rhinitis

Key points in the history would be:

- Itch of
    - palate
    - eyes
    - nose
    - throat
- Sneezing
- Watery nasal discharge

A searching history is needed to identify culpable allergens, e.g.

- House dust and house dust mite
- Pollens of grasses, trees and flowers
- Feathers and down
- Moulds and spores
- Animal dander

The symptoms of allergic rhinitis may be indistinguishable from vasomotor rhinitis.

Vasomotor rhinitis

This is exacerbated by:

- Perfume
- Sprays
- Change in air temperature
- Tobacco smoke and other pollutants

Also:

- Itch is not usually present
- Sides of blockage may alternate
- Vasomotor and allergic rhinitis may coexist
- Onset may be associated with hormonal changes of puberty and menopause
- Onset may be associated with anxiety and frustration; it is said that children cry through their eyes and adults through their noses!

Nasal polypi

These produce a more steady development of symptoms and may be an extension of allergic or vasomotor rhinitis. Also the patient may have:

- Had previous polypectomies
- Diminution or loss of sense of smell

FINDINGS IN RHINITIS EITHER ALLERGIC OR VASOMOTOR

- Swollen inferior turbinates (Fig. 13.1)
- Pale or mauve coloured inferior turbinates
- Moist nasal mucosa
- Allergic crease from repeated allergic 'salutes' which are more obvious in young people (Fig. 13.2)
- Reduced nasal airway

To distinguish between allergic and vasomotor rhinitis, the history is often more helpful than relying on specific physical findings.

Skin tests

Now difficult to obtain because of restrictions on hyposensitizing regimes; there must be full resuscitation facilities on site and the patient must remain for 2 h in those conditions. The scope for skin tests in general practice is very limited and most often not practicable. The skin test solutions are, therefore, not considered commercially viable by most of the manufacturers and are difficult to obtain as a result.

RAST (radioabsorbent sensitivity test) is readily available although expensive and is performed on a sample of venous blood.

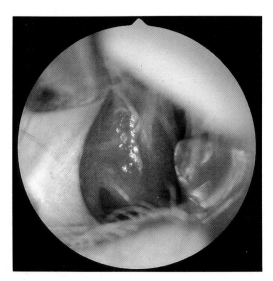

Fig. 13.1   Swollen inferior turbinates are often a cause of nasal blockage because of their allergic and non-allergic mucosal congestion.

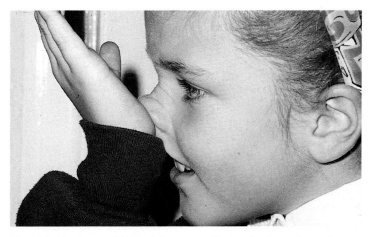

Fig. 13.2 Persistent rubbing of the nose to alleviate the discomfort and momentarily improve the airflow. This will eventually cause a crease of the skin on the nasal bridge.

MANAGEMENT OF ALLERGIC AND VASOMOTOR RHINITIS

(1) Topical medications

These are the treatment of choice:

- Intra-nasal steroid sprays; if the powder form of spray medication causes crusting and scanty bleeding, convert to an aqueous form, e.g. beclomethasone (Beconase), budesonide (Rhinocort), flunisolide (Syntaris).

- Avoidance advice concerning likely allergens.

- If nasal drip predominates, topical anticholinergic spray such as ipratropium (Rinatec) may be helpful.

- If cacosmia or facial pain occurs, a sinus X-ray should be done to exclude **paranasal sepsis** before starting intra-nasal steroids.

(2) Oral treatment

We have found oral medications to be more useful to support topical intra-nasal treatment. In cases of residual nasal or additional extra-nasal symptoms, then oral medications can be strongly recommended:

- Antihistamines, e.g. astemizole (Hismanal), terfenadine (Triludan)
- Pseudoephedrine may help in vasomotor rhinitis
- Combination preparations combining an antihistamine and a sympathomimetic

(3) Inhalation

- Steam (not directly from kettle)
- Menthol
- Tinct benzoin

These inhalations reduce the discomfort of nasal blockage and can be taken for a few minutes every 2 h.

(4) Surgery

Surgery to reduce the size of the inferior turbinates is strongly advised when:

- Blockage is severe
- Medical treatment fails

Surgical reduction of inferior turbinates will improve both patency as well as access for future topical intra-nasal steroids.

MANAGEMENT OF NASAL POLYPI (Fig. 13.3) IN GENERAL PRACTICE

- If symptoms mild, intra-nasal steroid drops, e.g. beclomethasone (Betnesol drops), should be applied twice a day with the head in the extended position. Regular steroid sprays may be preferred and worth trying as an alternative to drops. A sinus X-ray should be done to exclude fluid levels. Minimal mucosal thickening can be accepted. Smoking should be discouraged.

REFER when:

- Medical management fails
- Severe blockage at initial presentation
- Neoplasm suspected by the presence of a unilateral polyp with or without bleeding
- Nasal polyps are often recurrent, and in such cases, the patient will require maintenance intra-nasal steroid spray

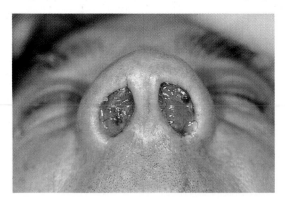

Fig. 13.3   Nasal polyps usually arise from the middle meatus.

SEPTAL DEVIATION

- May be associated with external deformity of either the nasal bridge or nasal tip or, indeed, both (Fig. 13.4)
- There may be a history of trauma, although not necessarily so
- Unilateral blockage is the presenting symptom
- May be coexistent with any of the aforementioned mucosal abnormalities

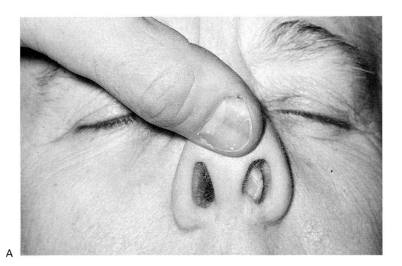

A

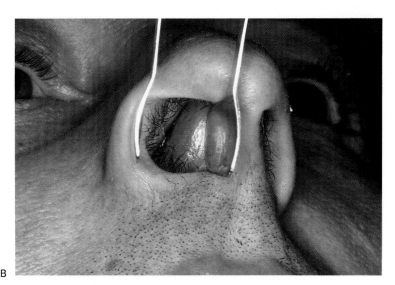

B

Fig. 13.4   The septal cartilage can be deviated at the **A** front or **B** middle.

Findings

- Tilting the nasal tip upwards by the clinician may reveal a deviation anteriorly or further back or indeed both.

- Reduced unilateral flow.

Management

- If blockage solely due to septal deviation REFER.

- If overlying allergic or non-allergic rhinitis, topical steroid sprays may just prove sufficient; if not REFER.

VALVULAR INSPIRATORY COLLAPSE

A minor degree of valvular movement of the nostrils during inspiration is physiologically normal. When excessive, the patient will present with nasal blockage on inspiration (Fig. 13.5). REFER

NASOPHARYNGEAL

Causes of obstruction are:

- Enlarged adenoids in children.

- Antrochoanal polyp hanging into nasopharynx; usually solitary.

- Tumours.

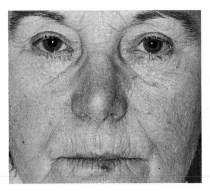 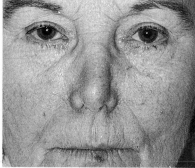

Fig. 13.5   Pronounced sucking in of the alae (nostrils) on inspiration reduces the airflow.

Management of suspected nasopharyngeal blockage

- If adenoids are thought to be responsible, have a lateral X-ray of the nasopharynx performed. If the air shadow is thicker than the soft palate shadow, adenoid enlargement is unlikely to be a major contribution to the blockage; if the air shadow is thinner than the soft palate shadow (Fig. 13.6) REFER.

- In both children and adults, check ears of secretary otitis media, as this may be due to eustachian tube obstruction caused by nasopharyngeal masses.

- Palpate the neck thoroughly in adults to exclude clinically enlarged cervical lymph nodes from a nasopharyngeal carcinoma.

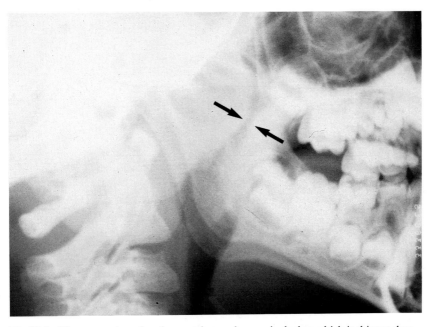

Fig. 13.6 The arrows show that the nasopharynx has an air shadow which is thinner than the soft palate; adenoid enlargement is the usual cause in children.

PITFALLS

- Rhinitis medicamentosa arises from prolonged use of non-steroidal topical applications which should, therefore, be avoided. The nasal mucosa swells to cause blockage as a result of these prolonged applications; further dosage, although relieving the blockage temporarily, causes further swelling, etc. If the patient has presented with blockage after self-medication REFER as these cases may require surgical help.

- Unilateral nasal discharge in children is a foreign body until otherwise proven; unless the foreign body is obvious at the nasal vestibule, in which case it can be hooked out, REFER URGENTLY.

- Children should not be diagnosed as having polyps except in cystic fibrosis; swollen inferior turbinates are often mistaken for polypi.

- The word 'catarrh' is nebulous and should not be used.

- Immigrant patients from hot climates (with relatively sparse fomites) may take a couple of years to show symptoms of house-dust allergy.

- A unilateral nasal polyp in the adult, with or without bleeding, should be REFERRED to exclude an underlying neoplasm.

- For long-term intra-nasal steroid maintenance treatment, drops should be avoided to prevent significant systemic absorption; the sprays should be used instead.

- Be aware of the valvular component in nasal blockage.

14. Epistaxis

Patients usually present with recurrent bleeding, often spontaneous, from one or both nostrils. Trauma causing nose bleeds may present to the GP, but more frequently attends an Accident and Emergency Department.

CHILDREN

- Children tend to bleed from varicose vessels over the anterior part of the septum known as the Little's area; i.e. that which can be seen when the nasal tip is tilted upwards (Fig. 14.1).
- Bleeding may be associated with:
  — coryza
  — exacerbation of allergic rhinitis
  — nose-picking
  — vestibulitis
  — foreign body associated with foul discharge
  — may be prodromal to exanthematous infections.

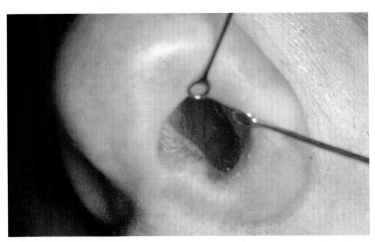

Fig. 14.1 Little's area is that area of the septum seen through the nostrils when the nasal tip is tilted upwards; anastomotic vessels in this area are prone to become varicose and bleed.

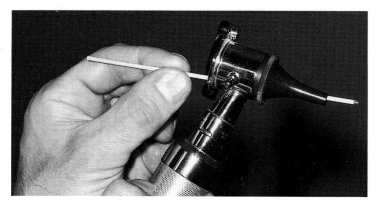

Fig. 14.2 The auriscope with a wide speculum provides magnification and light for chemical cautery to Little's area; the lens is swung to the side to allow access.

Management

- Bleeds from Little's area can normally be arrested by pinching the nasal vestibules by a parent or teacher. This should be associated with leaning forward to prevent blood entering the post-nasal space.

- Cauterize with silver nitrate sticks nitrate sticks after 5 min application of 4% lignocaine on cottonwool (Fig. 14.2). This should be followed by local application of an antibiotic/antiseptic cream; i.e. Naseptin/Vibrocil for 5–7 days.

- If no vessel is apparent because of slough or crusting over Little's area, then apply Naseptin cream for one week, then review.

- If there is no obvious bleeding point, consider blood dyscrasia or diathesis.

- For repeated bleeds REFER .

ADULTS

- Anterior bleeds from Little's area; treat as for children above.
- Posterior bleeds; these are suspected if no bleeding point can be seen anteriorly and cannot be stopped by pinching the nose.

Posterior bleeds:
- — occur more often in later life
- — are more severe in hypertension
- — may stop spontaneously
- — often present to the Accident and Emergency Department where the nose may be packed and the patient admitted.

Management

- Anterior bleeds
    - — treat with silver nitrate cautery and Naseptin (as per children).

- Posterior bleeds
    - — check blood pressure
    - — if recurrent REFER.
    - — if an intra-nasal mass is visible REFER.

PITFALLS

- Check to see if the patient is on anticoagulants or aspirin-based drugs.

- Check for signs of thrombocytopaenia and bleeding diatheses: REFER to haematologist.

- In young and adolescent males angiofibroma should be considered if substantial nasal blockage is present. REFER if no obvious bleeding from the septum.

15. Sinusitis

This diagnosis is frequently suspected in general practice. The following symptoms and signs are suggestive of sinusitis at initial presentation:

- Cacosmia
- Facial + frontal pain and tenderness
- Nasal blockage
- Mucopurulent rhinorrhoea
- Feverishness associated with above

Peri-orbital or frontal swellings (Pott's puffy tumour) may complicate sinusitis when infection is unchecked or inadequately treated; this scenario is unusual nowadays.

Associated constitutional symptoms in sinusitis may be:

- Sensation of congestion in face, head and ears
- Light-headedness

On this basis, it would be reasonable to treat this initial presentation as an acute **rhino-sinusitis.**

MANAGEMENT

- If peri-orbital and frontal swellings, REFER to ENT department.

- The anaerobic environment within the infected sinus calls for the use of metronidazole (Flagyl); penicillin or erythromycin (Erythroped) should be added to deal with aerobic pathogens.

- Analgesics.

- Menthol and steam inhalations reduce the discomfort of nasal blockage.

- Should resolution fail REFER .

RECURRENT RHINO-SINUSITIS

Management

- Sinuses should be X-rayed to support or refute an underlying chronic sinus abnormality. The views requested by the general practitioner should be occipito-mental (to show maxillary antra) (Fig. 15.1A) and occipito-frontal (to show frontal sinuses and ethmoid cells).

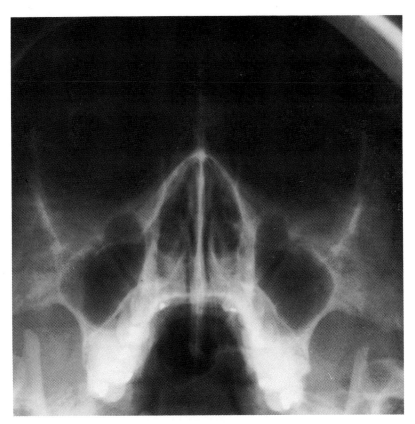

Fig. 15.1   A Normal OM view of maxillary sinus.

- If minimal mucosal thickening without fluid levels is seen on the X-ray (Fig. 15.1B), a working diagnosis of rhinitis, rather than sinusitis, should be considered (see Chapter 13).

- If fluid levels (Fig. 15.1C) or total opacities are shown, this should be treated as sinusitis.

- Bony erosion is suggestive of malignancy and should be REFERRED .

- Small mucosal cysts within the maxillary antra are not clinically important.

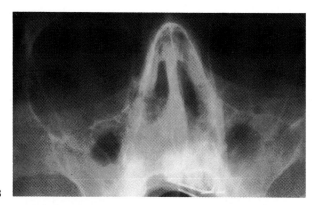

B

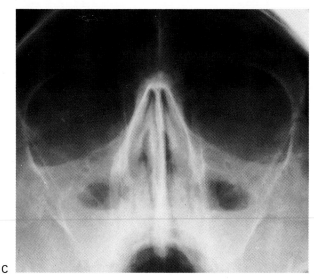

C

Fig. 15.1   B Maxillary mucosal thickening seen as an OM view.
C Fluid level.

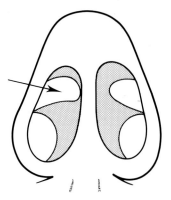

Fig. 15.2 Middle turbinate impaction on the septum.

- In the absence of any radiographic abnormality, the diagnosis of sinusitis is highly unlikely. The clinician should, therefore, look for the source of referred pain. Nasal turbinate impaction onto the septum is the most likely (Fig. 15.2) REFER.

Treatment

This can be classified into:

(1)   Those cases whom the GP can help

- Acute exacerbations of a recurrent infective picture require the use of:
    — metronidazole to cover likely anaerobes as well as erythromycin or penicillin
    — analgesics
    — menthol and steam inhalations may reduce the discomfort of nasal blockage.

- Allergic rhinitis (see Chapter 13). Intra-nasal steroid sprays are often useful. If steroid sprays fail because of poor nasal patency, such patients need REFERRAL for inferior turbinate shrinkage. Intra-nasal steroids are contra-indicated where there is radiographic evidence of paranasal sepsis; REFER for diagnostic washout.

- Small nasal polypi may respond to intra-nasal sprays or intra-nasal steroid drops, provided the sinus X-rays are either clear or show minimal mucosal thickening (see Chapter 13).

(2) Those cases requiring $\boxed{REFERRAL}$

- Recurrent infections should be $\boxed{\text{REFERRED}}$ for further assessment and possible surgery on the lateral nasal wall using modern endoscopic equipment
- Large nasal polypi for excision
- Gross septal deviations
- Suspected antro-ethmoidal carcinoma

PITFALLS

- Post-nasal drip alone is a non-specific symptom and is often environmentally related.

- In uncomplicated sinusitis, facial swelling does not occur. Facial swelling and tenderness indicate dental abscess, $\boxed{\text{REFER}}$ to dental practitoner.

- Facial expansion with ipsilateral blood-stained nasal discharge may represent a neoplasm; check for proptosis, cheimosis, palatal expansion and diminished hemi-palatal sensation on that side.

- Peri-orbital cellulitis presenting (in children especially) implies that sinusitis has progressed into the anterior peri-orbital tissue via the ethmoid cells. $\boxed{\text{REFER}}$ for parenteral antibiotic treatment as an in-patient.

- Frontal swellings in relation to a suspected diagnosis of sinusitis should be $\boxed{\text{REFERRED}}$ to exclude frontal osteomyelitis, mucocele or large osteoma.

- Rhinitis medicamentosa can be avoided by restricting intra-nasal medications to steroidal types.

16. Sore throat

This is a frequently presenting symptom of many mild conditions associated with upper respiratory tract viruses which often may require simple management.

(1) PHARYNGITIS

This is characterized by some or all of the following:

- Sore or dry throat
- Worse in morning
- No constitutional disturbance
- Patient may be aware of nasal obstruction, especially at night
- Associated coryza

(2) TONSILLITIS

This is diagnosed from the history:

- Sore throat and swollen tonsils associated with
  — severe malaise
  — pyrexia
  — recurrent cervical lymphadenopathy
  — referred earache
  — halitosis

(3) PERITONSILLAR CELLULITIS

This is the pre-suppurative stage of quinsy and always develops from tonsillitis and will also show:

- Unilateral peritonsillar swelling and redness
- Relatively little trismus

(4) QUINSY

This is the next stage and represents a localized collection of pus above the tonsil. The features are:

- Those of peritonsillar cellulitis
- Trismus (spasm of pterygoid muscles preventing opening of the mouth)

FINDINGS

Appearance of tonsils between attacks of tonsillitis is not helpful unless they are so big as to cause dysphagia or airway obstruction during sleep (see below).

During an attack of sore throat of **viral origin** there may be:

- Generalized mucosal injection with or without ulceration
- If ulceration of palate or pharynx is unilateral, consider herpes zoster (Ramsay-Hunt)
- Palatal petechiae
- Uvular oedema
- Cold sores (herpes simplex I) on lips or nostrils

Tonsillitis may show:

- Aggressive injection and swelling limited to the tonsils and faucial pillars.
- Crypts full of *pus* suggestive, but not diagnostic, of tonsillitis; crypts can contain pus even when quiescent.
- Foetor
- 'Plummy speech'
- Facial flushing
- Pyrexia
- Tender cervical lymphadenopathy
- General malaise

Glandular fever (syn infectious mononucleosis) may show:

- Foetor
- 'Plummy speech'
- Slough on grossly swollen tonsils (Fig. 16.1)
- Palatal petechiae
- Pyrexia
- LKKS and general lymphadenopathy
- General malaise

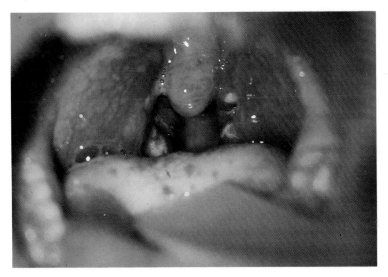

Fig. 16.1   Slough on tonsils as seen in glandular fever.

MANAGEMENT OF SORE THROAT

- Sore throats without trismus benefit from aspirin gargles (only for adults) and analgesics.

- The majority of patients with sore throats have probably managed themselves for a day or so with simple analgesics before presenting themselves ot the GP's surgery.

- At this stage, if a diagnosis of tonsillitis is made, oral antibiotics can be started, preferably cefuroxime axetil (Zinnat) phenoxymethylpenicillin or erythromycin (Erythroped) for 10 days. It has been shown that a 10 days course (as opposed to 5–7 days) reduces the incidence of recurrence. Ampicillin-based drugs should be avoided if glandular fever is suspected. If therapy fails   REFER .

- If frequency and severity of tonsillitis is causing concern to the patient or parent of affected child, despite medical treatment   REFER .

MANAGEMENT OF GLANDULAR FEVER

- Constitutional disturbance does not respond to antibiotics.

- Prolonged periods of rest will be required and the condition may take months to settle, waxing and waning as it does so; this should be explained to the patient.

- Subtle changes in liver function tests are common but clinically overt liver dysfunction is rare.

- Monospot and film are advised to check diagnosis about a week after onset.

- Superadded depression may require separate treatment.

MANAGEMENT OF RECURRENT OR CHRONIC PHARYNGITIS

- Check nasal patency; chronic mouth-breathing will dry and irritate the throat.

- Check sinus X-ray to exclude paranasal sepsis; REFER if sinuses are opaque, show fluid levels or have gross mucosal thickening.

- If sinus X-rays are clear or show minimal mucosal thickening, start either oral decongestants or intra-nasal steroid spray; both modalities may be needed.

- Discourage smoking and chronic use of proprietary throat lozenges or sprays.

- If the pharyngitis secondary to nasal obstruction has not responded to oral decongestants or intra-nasal steroids REFER.

OTHER CAUSES

- Iatrogenic from prolonged antibiotics for other disorders resulting in candidal pharyngitis (Fig. 16.2)
- NSAID usage causing agranulocytosis
- Gross dental caries; requires dental REFERRAL
- Tobacco
- Gastro-oesophageal reflux of acid/bile
- Alcohol overuse
- Occupational irritants
- Voice abuse; consider speech therapy REFERRAL
- Styloid pain is elicited by palpating the tonsil on the affected side with a gloved finger. REFER
- Venereal disease

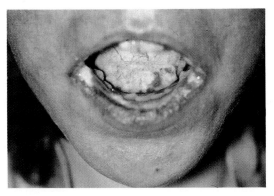

Fig. 16.2   An extreme example of oral candidiasis. This tongue is infected with Candida, which can extend to the pharynx.

PITFALLS

- Unilaterally sore or enlarged tonsil, in the absence of acute inflammation, is strongly suggestive of neoplasia. REFER

- Ampicillin-based drugs as first-line treatment should not be used in suspected glandular fever because a rash can be induced ('poor man's monospot'!).

- Recurrent generalized pharyngitis with worsening debility should prompt a blood film to exclude leukaemia.

17. Hoarseness

This is an abnormality of the voice affecting:

- Pitch
- Volume
- Resonance
- Quality

Hoarseness is often associated with an URTI in the otherwise healthy patient; these are mostly of viral origin.

MANAGEMENT

- Limit the use of the voice to quiet conversation.

- Analgesic if associated sore throat.

- Steam inhaled from a mixture of hot water and benzoin tincture (5 ml in one pint of hot water).

- Patients with hoarseness that fails to resolve in 2 weeks should be REFERRED to exclude neoplasia, nodules or vocal polypi.

FURTHER POINTS OF HISTORY

- Weight-loss suggestive of upper or lower respiratory tract cancer. REFER

- Weight-gain suggestive of myxoedema. Investigate and treat. REFER if hoarseness persists.

- Associated dysphagia is suggestive of upper respiratory cancer and palsies of the larynx or pharynx; REFER.

- Referred earache may be an associated symptom of an underlying respiratory tract neoplasm.

- Neck swellings suggest cervical lymphadenopathy, possibly associated with underlying neoplasia.

- History of contributory suppurative disease
  — sinusitis
  — bronchitis
  — bronchiectasis.

- History of dyspepsia and gastro-oesophageal reflux.

- Chemical trauma.
  — industrial
  — smoking.

- Voice abuse can result in the use of the false vocal cords or nodules on the true cords.

MANAGEMENT

This is dependent on the treatment of the causative illness, occupation or habit. ENT REFERRAL is often mandatory for exclusion of malignancy.

18. Dysphagia

This is difficulty in swallowing (aphagia means inability to swallow) either fluids, solids or both.

POINTS OF HISTORY

(a) Acute

Cases with constitutional disturbance are usually inflammatory:

- Supraglottitis (formerly known as epiglottitis); must be REFERRED urgently
- Tonsillitis causing pain, obstruction or both (see Chapter 16)
- Quinsy REFER
- Glandular fever; may need REFERRAL for intravenous hydration and steroids if severe

Foreign bodies tend to present to the Accident and Emergency Department, but if suspected, REFER URGENTLY.

(b) Progressive

Cases should arouse suspicion of **pharyngeal** or **oesophageal neoplasia**:

- History of weight-loss and fatigue
- Usually progressively worsening dysphagia for solids to semi-solids to liquids in that order
- Hoarseness
- Cough on drinking suggests aspiration

History suggestive of a benign cause of progressive dysphagia

- Regurgitation of recognizable food suggests a pharyngeal pouch (Fig. 18.1). Do a barium swallow to confirm and REFER.

- Long-standing acid reflux suggests peptic stricture at the lower end of the oesophagus. REFER to surgical or medical colleague.

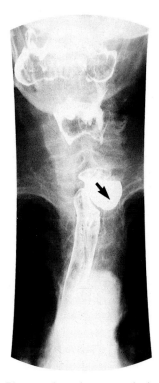

Fig. 18.1   Pharyngeal pouch seen on a barium swallow.

Other problems

- Neurogenic dysphagia may be associated with nasal escape because of palatal paresis along with other cranial nerve palsies. This situation suggests a neoplasm (either primary or secondary) at the base of the skull or a specific neurological condition, e.g. bulbar palsy.

- Connective tissue disorder, e.g. systemic sclerosis.

(c)   Prolonged and variable 'lump in throat'

Without constitutional disturbance, this is suggestive of **globus pharyngeus** (formerly known as globus hystericus). The term **pseudodysphagia** is the most satisfactory; this presents a difficult diagnostic problem:

- History of a 'lump in throat' which tends to be relieved by the act of swallowing, only to return soon after.

- The 'lump' is variable.

- No constitutional disturbance.

- There may be an anxiety element because the patient fears the diagnosis of cancer; a relative, friend or neighbour may have had such a diagnosis.

These patients should be REFERRED for clinical and endoscopic examination.

POINTS OF EXAMINATION

General examination
- Pallid complexion
- Evidence of weight-loss
- Abdominal masses
- Chest findings suggesting secondary infections or consolidations associated with aspiration and chest neoplasm
- Cranial and peripheral nervous system if applicable

Local examination
- Angular cheilitis
- Glossitis
- Neck masses
- Oral masses
    — mouth
    — retromolar trigone (see glossary)
    — oropharynx (the rest of the pharynx will be examined in the ENT Department)

- Movements of
    — tongue
    — palate
    — pharynx

- Sensory examination of palate and pharynx

MANAGEMENT

Investigations should include:

- Lateral soft tissue X-ray of neck
- Chest X-ray
- Barium swallow
- Full blood count and ESR

If neoplasia or neurogenic cause is suspected, $\boxed{\text{REFER}}$ with appropriate information.

19. The primary health care team

Most GP's are part of a team of health care workers. These people can help in the handling of ENT problems within the community.

The health care workers comprise:

THE PRACTICE NURSE

The practice nurse can be trained by the local ENT Department

- To perform ear syringing
- To introduce ½ inch ribbon gauze wicks into ears
- To arrest nose bleeds by squeezing the tip of the nose over the Little's area (Fig. 19.1)
- To perform audiograms if the practice has access to audiometry equipment
- To take blood samples and swabs where appropriate

THE HEALTH VISITOR

- Is often the primary contact with a parent who suspects a hearing problem in their baby
- Performs routine hearing tests

    (i) 0–6 months, 'startle' reflex
    (ii) 6–9 months, distraction test
    (iii) 16–30 months, co-operative test
    (iv) 3–5 years, toy discrimination test and pure-tone sweep frequency test

- Assesses speech and language development
- Arranges pure-tone audiometry for children at the local audiometry department

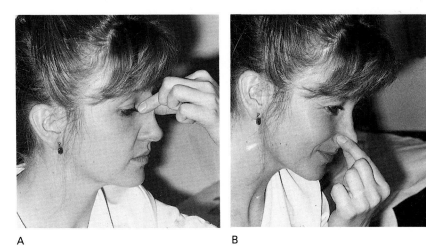

A   B

Fig. 19.1   (a) Pinching the bones will not stop a nose bleed. (b) Pinching the nasal vestibules onto the anterior septum will compress culpable vessels in Little's area.

THE DISTRICT NURSE

- Performs ear syringing at a patient's home
- Assists with the administration of medicine at a patient's home
- Performs tracheostomy care (Fig. 19.2)

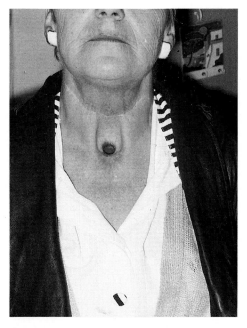

Fig. 19.2   This tracheostomy is part of a total laryngectomy.

THE SCHOOL MEDICAL OFFICER

- Performs primary and secondary school entry hearing tests.
- May well refer cases of suspected deafness to an ENT clinic whence correspondence will be sent to the GP.

PRIVATE HEARING CENTRES

- Some patients may self-refer to these services. The centre may send a report of their findings and actions to the GP.

20. The GP and ENT post-operative sequelae

Most post-operative care of ENT problems will be conducted by the ENT department. However, there are some ENT problems which, more often than not, present to the GP rather than the hospital department.

TONSILLECTOMY

Post-operative bleeding

Reactive bleeding takes place **within 48 h of tonsillectomy** and is due either to a ligature slipping or a vessel opening up spontaneously; as the patient is very likely to be in hospital at the time of this particular emergency, it is unlikely to be seen at home. **Emergency readmission to hospital** is clearly necessary.

Secondary bleeding

This occurs within **5–10 days** of the operation and the patient is likely to be at home. The traditional teaching is that secondary bleeding occurs as a result of an infection in the tonsillar fossae but there is little evidence to support this. More likely it is due to a piece of granulation tissue having separated. The patient should be **referred back urgently to the ENT department** where admission will be arranged for a day or two for careful observation with or without antibiotic treatment depending on the policy of the particular surgeon. Secondary bleeding is usually less brisk than reactive bleeds.

Post-operative pain

Although the patient is usually released from hospital with suitable oral analgesia, post-operative throat pain, including referred earache, often gets worse three days or so post-operatively once the patient is at home (Fig. 20.1). The GP is sometimes called at this point; a common error is to misconstrue normal proteinaceous exudate for pus and infection. If **post-operative antibiotics** were started post-operatively by the ENT department as a matter of policy, this drug will be substituted for another in the mistaken belief of an infection. The patient is usually apyrexial and will respond well to the addition of **soluble aspirin gargles 600 mg qds** and swallowed. Aspirin may not be desirable in the immediate post-operative period because of increased incidence of haemorrhage. **Aspirin must not be given to children; use a paracetamol mucilage or syrup.** Recent work has shown intramuscular diclofenac to be helpful; this does not interfere with platelet action. Up to two intramuscular injection of 75 mg on successive days can be used, but no more than this. The cause of the late pain reaction is the leisurely deposition of post-traumatic inflammatory substances. In the unlikely event of a pyrexia, then infection should be clearly considered. Although **earache** is usually referred, the tympanic membranes should nevertheless be examined to exclude an otitis media. Temporomandibular joint pain is most unusual in this context.

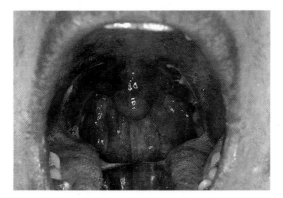

Fig. 20.1   Postoperative slough in the tonsillar fossae.

General points

In the midst of distress, the adult patient or the parent of a young patient may regret the whole business of having submitted to the operation; careful explanation and encouragement that after 2 weeks, everything will have settled, are necessary. As far as **food** is concerned, rough food, such as nuts, crisps and fruit, little and often, will help keep the throat clean and the underlying muscles active; battling with one or two large meals a day should be discouraged, as should languishing with ice-creams and jellies.

ADENOIDECTOMY

Post-operative bleeding

Post-nasal bleeding into the mouth should prompt **urgent readmission** with a view to post-nasal packing.

Post-operative pain

Post-operative pain after adenoidectomy is minimal, if at all. Referred earache should not be diagnosed until the tympanic membranes have been examined to exclude otitis media.

GROMMETS

The GP will sometimes be consulted about a **discharge** from an ear which has recently had a grommet inserted. This may occur as a result of an URTI or contamination, such as swimming-bath water.

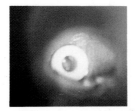

Fig. 20.2   This grommet is ventilating the middle ear via the lumen through which the middle ear mucosa can be seen. The colour of the grommet material will vary according to the manufacturer.

A 5-day course of **antibiotic ear drops** should clear this or at least improve matters. Should this fail, the patient should be sent to the ENT department for further evaluation; more likely than not, the grommet will have to be removed at that stage.

Parents will nearly all ask whether their child can **swim with grommets**. There is now evidence to show that children with grommets who swim do not have any more trouble than those who have been forbidden. Advice will still vary from surgeon to surgeon but sensible advice would be to advocate some form of ear plug and avoidance of ducking and diving. This topic will usually be covered in the ENT department. Shampoos and conditioners in the ears should also be avoided.

NASAL SURGERY

Pain

Pain is unusual post-operatively. Nasal splints which are inserted to pre-vent the formation of adhesions may occasionally cause distressing pain; this is due to the pressure of the splints or the suture used to secure the splints. If there are no obvious signs of infection, analgesics will help. If there is **swelling or gross infection of the nasal tip,** the patient should be **referred back to the ENT department.**

Epistaxis

Epistaxis should be redirected to the ENT department. Blood-staining of mucous discharge is usually a reaction to surgical trauma and will soon settle.

The use of cottonwool to wipe the nose rather than paper tissues will help prevent a frictional vestibulitis of the nose; an **antibiotic cream,** such as Naseptin, is a useful adjunct and should be used for 5 days.

21. Glossary of specialist vocabulary commonly used in correspondence from ENT departments

This list is clearly not comprehensive of all the specialist terms, some of which will be used within the realms of other specialities and will therefore be more widely known.

Acoustic neuroma: A Schwannoma of the vestibular division of the auditory nerve; this is benign, although pressure symptoms render it life-threatening if the tumour is large.

Anosmia: Lack of sense of smell.

Antrostomy: A commonly used term for an intra-nasal antrostomy, which is the creation of a large hole between the nasal cavity and the ipsilateral maxillary sinus. This is gradually being superseded by functional endoscopic sinus surgery.

Audiogram: A *pure-tone audiogram* is a chart of the pure-tone thresholds at various frequencies. A *speech audiogram* is a graph illustrating the ability of the subject to discriminate between similarly sounding words and may be used in conjunction with other tests to differentiate between a cochlear and auditory nerve deafness.

Brain stem evoked response: A measure of auditory pathway electrical activity in response to clicking sounds. This is an objective test, over which the patient has no control, as opposed to pure-tone and speech audiometry where the patient's subjective response is recorded.

Cacosmia: A subjective unpleasant smell.

Cageusia: A bad taste in the mouth.

Caldwell-Luc: A surgical approach to the maxillary antrum via an incision above the upper canine and pre-molar teeth. Once the antrum is entered, irreversibly inflamed mucosa can be stripped away. An intra-nasal antrostomy is usually done at the same time to allow easy access to wash out post-operative blood clots and debris.

Caloric test: The assessment of labyrinthine function by warm and cold fluid application to the tympanic membrane; in cases of tympanic perforation, cold and warm air is used. The duration of the resulting nystagmus is recorded and compared one side with the other. A conclusion can, therefore, be drawn as to whether a particular labyrinth is paretic.

Choanal atresia: A congenital absence of a posterior nasal passageway; this can be either unilateral or bilateral.

Cholesteatoma: An encysted collection of squamous epithelial debris, usually originating in the upper reaches of the middle ear and often involving the mastoid antrum.

Crico-pharyngeal myotomy: Surgical splitting of the crico-pharyngeus muscle at the top of the oesophagus, performed either internally or externally. When performed internally through an endoscope, it is often referred to as Dohlman's operation.

Cricothyrotomy: A surgically produced hole in the crico-thyroid membrane as an alternative to a tracheostomy, in order to relieve upper respiratory obstruction.

Dohlman's operation: An endoscopic approach to performing crico-pharyngeal myotomy using diathermy.

Dysarthria: Incoordinate enunciation of speech.

Dysphasia: A disorder of symbolic function of speech, distorting understanding and verbal expression.

Dysphonia: Abnormality of pitch, volume, resonance or quality of voice.

Electrocochleogram: An objective measurement of electrical activity of the cochlea in response to clicking sounds. In children, this usually requires a short general anaesthetic.

Epiglottitis: A clinical emergency arising from an acute inflammation and oedema of the epiglottis and surrounding supraglottic tissues; the term supraglottitis is now more commonly used.

Ethmoiditis: Inflammation of the ethmoid cells, thought to be largely responsible for the formation of nasal polyps.

Functional endoscopic sinus surgery: The use of rigid fibre-optic telescopes is taking on increasing importance; the concept is to restore sinus ventilation with minimum disruption to the lateral nasal wall – this is less traumatic than the older 'blunderbuss' treatments.

Furuncle: A boil of a hair follicle in the skin of the outer third of the external auditory meatus; the inner two-thirds of the canal skin does not contain hair follicles.

Globus syndrome: A sensation of a lump in the throat, without true dysphagia. The term globus hystericus is incorrect and has been superseded by two terms: globus pharyngeus and pseudodysphagia.

Glomus tumour: A tumour of baroreceptor tissue in (a) internal jugular vein, (b) middle ear, (c) the vagus nerve as it emerges from the skull.

Glossitis: Inflammation of the tongue.

Glossodynia: Painful tongue; this symptom may not have any demonstrable physical basis.

Glottis: Synonymous with the true vocal cords. The area above is called the supraglottis and the area below the subglottis.

Glue ear: A term often used for an effusion in the middle ear whose synonyms are serous otitis media, otitis media with effusion, secretory otitis media and catarrhal otitis.

Herpes zoster oticus: A herpes zoster infection of the geniculate ganglion in the temporal bone, causing ipsilateral facial palsy and painful rash of the external ear, palate, pharynx and rarely the larynx. There may be associated sensori-neural deafness. The term Ramsay-Hunt syndrome is used synonymously.

Incudo-stapedial joint: The joint of articulation between the long process of incus and the head of stapes. It can be disrupted by chronic retraction of the tympanic membrane over the joint, chronic suppurative otitis media, recurrent acute otitis media and trauma, either accidental or surgical.

Inverted papilloma: Otherwise known as transitional cell papilloma, arising from nasal or sinus mucosa. Rarely pre-malignant.

Keratosis obturans: An accumulation of debris in the deep part of the external auditory canal causing painful erosion of the surrounding bone, thought to be due to defective epithelial migration along the external auditory canal.

Laryngocele: An abnormal herniation of the laryngeal mucosa between true and false cords. This may well present with a lump in the neck, worsened by blowing against a resistance, e.g. trumpets. Swelling can appear externally, internally in the valleculae or both.

Laryngomalacia: Synonymously known as a floppy larynx which is a self-curing infantile condition presenting with stridor.

Lermoyez syndrome: A variant of Ménière's syndrome, where tinnitus and deafness are relieved by the onset of vertigo.

Leukoplakia: Literally, a white patch caused by dysplastic or early malignant squamous epithelium.

Ludwig's angina: Cellulitis of the floor of the mouth and neck, caused by haemolytic streptococcus.

Mastoidectomy: An operation to remove diseased mastoid bone. A *radical mastoidectomy* is performed in the management of cholesteatoma. A *modified radical mastoidectomy* is a radical mastoidectomy with preservation or reconstruction of parts of the ossicles and tympanic membrane. A *cortical mastoidectomy* is performed for mucosal disease and is less commonly used than formerly.

Ménière's syndrome: A quartet of symptoms; prodromal sensation of fullness in the ear, along with vertigo which is associated with variable hearing and tinnitus. The syndrome is the clinical manifestation of Ménière's disease which encompasses the syndrome with the known microscopic abnormalities of the cochlea.

Myringitis: Inflammation, usually granular or bullous, specifically of the tympanic membrane.

Myringostome: A less commonly used synonym for a tympanic membrane perforation.

Myringotomy: A small incision made in the tympanic membrane to release middle ear fluid; this incisional site allows insertion of a grommet.

Nystagmus: Involuntary oscillation of the eyes, having two components: slow and fast. The slow phase is due to the labyrinth disorder itself and the fast phase is due to cortical correction. By convention, it is the direction of the fast phase which is used to label the direction of nystagmus.

Osler's syndrome: A foreshortened term which should really include the names of Weber and Rendu, synonymous with hereditary telangectasia and often presenting with epistaxis.

Otorrhagia: Specifically bleeding from the ear.

Otorrhoea: The general term for discharge from the ear; this word should be qualified by the type of discharge, e.g. mucous.

Otosclerosis: A proliferation of bone derived from the otic capsule; in practical terms, otosclerosis applies to an area of proliferation of bone around the stapes foot-plate.

Ozaena: An unpleasant smell emanating from the nose due to atrophic rhinitis. The smell is noticed by those around, although uncommonly by the sufferer because of damage to the olfactory epithelium.

Pharyngeal pouch: Synonymous with hypopharyngeal pouch and Zenker's diverticulum. An abnormal herniation of mucosa between a thyro-pharyngeus and a crico-pharyngeus in the lower reaches of the pharynx.

Polyp: A macroscopic term regardless of histology, to describe a pedun-culated mass, not necessarily neoplastic, attached to a surface. A nasal polyp really represents herniated mucosa and oedema from the lateral nasal wall; an aural polyp represents granulation tissue although present-ing macroscopically in a polypoid shape.

Presbycusis: The wear and tear of the cochlear hair cells.

Quinsy: An abscess (localized collection of pus) above the tonsil.

Rannula: A mucosal cystic swelling in the floor of the mouth.

Reinke's oedema: Swelling of both vocal cords due to sub-epithelial oedema.

Retromolar trigone: Area in the mouth between the lower back teeth and side of tongue; exposed clinically by retracting the tongue away from the teeth.

Rhinorrhoea: A nasal discharge; the term should be qualified by the qual-ity of discharge, e.g. watery.

Sialadenitis: Inflammation of the salivary glands.

Stridor: Abnormal laryngeal sounds, specific to the respiratory cycle.

Supraglottis: The area of the larynx above the glottis or true vocal cords.

Subglottis: The area of the larynx below the glottis or true vocal cords.

Tracheostomy: A surgically fashioned hole from the exterior into the trachea, to relieve upper respiratory obstruction.

Tracheotomy: The surgical action of making the hole in the trachea.

Tympanoplasty: Surgical repair of middle ear sound conduction mechanism. In effect, a tympanoplasty is a myringoplasty with surgical attention to the ossicles as well.

Tympanosclerosis: Chalk patches deposited within the substance of the tympanic membrane as a result of inflammation which has organized. These chalk patches can also occur in the mucosa around the ossicles.

Tympanotomy: An incision in the posterior meatal wall to lift up the external auditory canal skin in continuity with the tympanic membrane so that the middle ear can be exposed for diagnostic inspection or surgical procedures. The incision is used, for example, in stapedectomy, where a plastic prosthesis is inserted in place of a fixed stapes bone.

Vertigo: A hallucination of rotatory movement; not to be confused with lighht-headedness.

Index